Nursing Facts

Facts

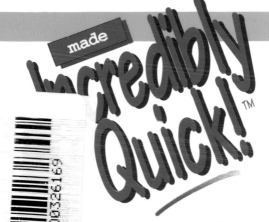

made

Incredibly

Quick!™

D0326169

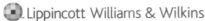

Lippincott Williams & Wilkins
a Wolters Kluwer business
Philadelphia · Baltimore · New York · London
Buenos Aires · Hong Kong · Sydney · Tokyo

Staff

Executive Publisher
Judith A. Schilling McCann, RN, MSN

Editorial Director
David Moreau

Clinical Director
Joan M. Robinson, RN, MSN

Senior Art Director
Arlene Putterman

Art Director
Mary Ludwicki

Senior Managing Editor
Tracy S. Diehl

Designer
Lynn Foulk

Illustrator
Bot Roda

Digital Composition Services
Diane Paluba (manager), Joyce Rossi Biletz

Associate Manufacturing Manager
Beth J. Welsh

Editorial Assistants
Megan L. Aldinger, Karen J. Kirk, Linda K. Ruhf

Indexer
Tracy S. Diehl

Vital signs, Cardiac, Respiratory, Neurologic, GI/GU, Musculoskeletal, Pain, Skin, Endocrine, Geriatric, Pediatric, Psychiatric

Panels: metabolic, lipid, thyroid; Chemistry; Tumor markers; CBC; Coagulation; Hematology; Antibiotics; Urine tests; Cardiac biomarkers; Crisis values; Acid-base

Calculations, Herb-drug interactions, Geriatric, Injections, Insulin, I.V.s, CVADs, Calculating drip rates, Ports, Med infusion rates

CPR, ACLS, Respiratory, Transfusion, Shock, ICP

Cardiac, Leads, Heart rate, Rhythm strips

Cancer, Heart valves and vessels, Respiratory and urinary tracts, GI system

Conversions, Precautions, Cultures, NANDA, Nutrition, Wounds, Eng.-Span., Abbrev., Weapons exposure

Assessment

Labs

Meds / I V

Emergency

ECG

Teaching

Resource

Abbreviations

ACT	activated clotting time	**MI**	myocardial infarction
AED	automated external defibrillator	**min**	minute
		ml	milliliter
AV	arterioventricular	**mm Hg**	millimeters of mercury
BP	blood pressure	**MS**	musculoskeletal
BUN	blood urea nitrogen	**neuro**	neurologic
cc	cubic centimeter	**NPH insulin**	neutral protamine Hagedorn insulin
CICU (CCU)	cardiac intensive care unit or coronary care unit	**NPO**	nothing by mouth
cm	centimeter	**NSR**	normal sinus rhythm
CNS	central nervous system	**OR**	operating room
CPR	cardiopulmonary resuscitation	**OT**	occupational therapy
		oz.	ounce
CV	cardiovascular	**PACU**	postanesthesia care unit
CVC	central vascular catheter	**PCA**	patient-controlled analgesia
D/C planning	discharge planning	**PEA**	pulseless electrical activity
ECG	electrocardiogram, electrocardiograph	**pH**	potential of hydrogen
		PMI	point of maximal impulse
ED	emergency department	**prn**	as needed
ET	endotracheal tube	**PT**	physical therapy; prothrombin time
ext.	extension		
g	gram	**PTT**	partial thromboplastin time
GI	gastrointestinal	**RBC**	red blood cell
gtt	drop	**resp.**	respiratory
GU	genitourinary	**RT**	respiratory therapy
HDL	high-density lipoprotein	S_1	first heart sound
hr.	hour	S_2	second heart sound
I&O	intake and output	S_3	third heart sound
IABP	intra-aortic balloon pump	S_4	fourth heart sound
ICP	intracranial pressure	**sec**	second(s)
ICU	intensive care unit	**SSRI**	selective serotonin reuptake inhibitor
I.M.	intramuscular		
INR	International Normalized Ratio	**stat**	immediately
IS	information service	**subQ**	subcutaneous
I.V.	intravenous	**tbs**	tablespoon
kg	kilogram	**TCA**	tricyclic antidepressant
L	liter	**trach**	tracheostomy
labs	laboratory results	**tsp**	teaspoon
lb.	pound	**VAP**	vascular access port
LDL	low-density lipoprotein	**VF**	ventricular fibrillation
m^2	meter squared	**VT**	ventricular tachycardia
MAOIs	monoamine oxidase inhibitors	**WBC**	white blood cell
mcg	microgram		
mg	milligram		

Vital signs

Vital-sign ranges vary from neonate to older adult, as shown in this chart.

Age	Temperature °F	Temperature °C	Pulse rate (beats/min)	Respiratory rate (breaths/min)	Blood pressure (mm Hg)
Neonate	98.6 to 99.8	37 to 37.7	110 to 160	30 to 50	73/45
3 years	98.5 to 99.5	36.9 to 37.5	80 to 125	20 to 30	90/55
10 years	97.5 to 98.6	36.4 to 37	70 to 110	16 to 22	96/57
16 years	97.6 to 98.8	36.4 to 37.1	55 to 100	15 to 20	120/80
Adult	96.8 to 99.5	36 to 37.5	60 to 100	12 to 20	120/80
Older adult	96.5 to 97.5	35.8 to 36.4	60 to 100	15 to 25	120/80

CARDIOVASCULAR SYSTEM

Cardiovascular assessment

Inspection
- No pulsations are visible except at point of maximum impulse (PMI).
- No lifts (heaves) or retractions are evident in four valve areas of chest wall.

Palpation
- No vibrations or thrills are evident.
- No lifts or heaves are evident.
- No pulsations are visible except at PMI and epigastric area.

Vascular palpation
- Note skin temperature, texture, and turgor.
- Capillary refill is no more than 3 seconds.
- Pulses should be regular in rhythm and strength.
  - 4+ = bounding
  - 3+ = increased
  - 2+ = normal
  - 1+ = weak
  - 0 = absent

Auscultation
- First heart sound (S_1) heard best with stethoscope diaphragm over mitral area.
- Second heart sound (S_2) heard best with stethoscope diaphragm over aortic area.
- Third heart sound (S_3) heard best with stethoscope bell over mitral area.
- Additional heart sound (S_4) heard best with stethoscope bell at mitral area.

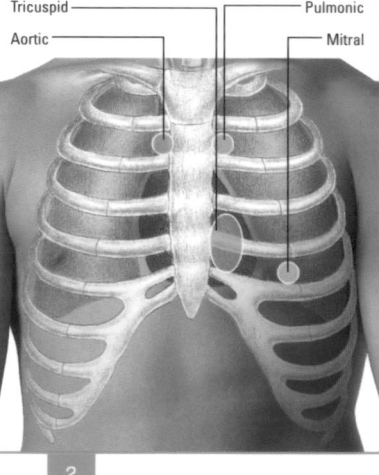

Heart sound sites

Tricuspid — Pulmonic

Aortic — Mitral

RESPIRATORY SYSTEM

Respiratory assessment

Inspection	Chest configuration, tracheal position, chest symmetry, skin condition, nostril flaring, accessory muscle use, respiratory rate and pattern, cyanosis, clubbing of fingers
Palpation	Crepitus, pain, tactile fremitus, scars, lumps, lesions, ulcerations, chest wall symmetry and expansion
Percussion	Resonance (normal), hyperresonance, dullness, tympany
Auscultation	Four types of breath sounds over normal lungs: Tracheal, bronchial, bronchovesicular, and vesicular

Abnormal breath sounds

Sound	Description
Crackles	Light cracking, popping, intermittent, nonmusical sounds; like hairs rubbed together; heard on inspiration or expiration
Pleural friction rub	Low-pitched, continual, superficial, squeaking or grating sound; like pieces of sandpaper being rubbed together; heard on inspiration and expiration
Rhonchi	Low-pitched, snoring, monophonic sounds heard primarily on expiration; may be heard throughout the respiratory cycle
Stridor	High-pitched, monophonic crowing sound heard on inspiration; louder in the neck than chest wall
Wheezes	High-pitched, continual, musical or whistling sound heard on expiration; may be heard on inspiration and expiration

Auscultation sequence

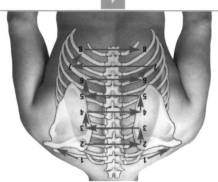

Anterior

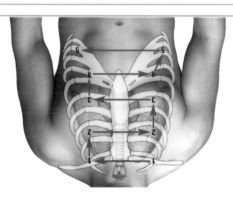

Posterior

4

Neurologic stages of altered arousal

This chart highlights the six stages of altered arousal. An alert patient responds to voice and has purposeful movement and appropriate spontaneous activity.

Stage	Manifestations
Confusion	• Loss of ability to think rapidly and clearly • Impaired judgment and decision making
Disorientation	• Beginning loss of consciousness • Disorientation to time progressing to disorientation to place • Impaired memory • Lack of recognition of self (last symptom)
Lethargy	• Limited spontaneous movement or speech • Easily aroused by normal speech or touch • Possible disorientation to time, place, or person
Obtundation	• Mild to moderate reduction in arousal • Limited responsiveness to environment • Ability to fall asleep easily without verbal or tactile stimulation • Minimum response to questions
Stupor	• State of deep sleep or unresponsiveness • Arousable with difficulty (motor or verbal response only to vigorous and repeated stimulation) • Withdrawal or grabbing response to stimulation
Coma	• Lack of motor or verbal response to external environment or stimuli • No response to noxious stimuli such as deep pain • Can't be aroused by any stimulus

Glasgow Coma Scale

A decreased score in one or more categories may signal an impending neurologic crisis. The best response is scored.

Test	Score	Patient's response
Eye opening		
Spontaneously	4	Opens eyes spontaneously
To speech	3	Opens eyes to verbal command
To pain	2	Opens eyes to painful stimulus
None	1	Doesn't open eyes in response to stimulus
Motor response		
Obeys	6	Reacts to verbal command
Localizes	5	Identifies localized pain
Withdraws	4	Flexes and withdraws from painful stimulus
Abnormal flexion	3	Assumes a decorticate position
Abnormal extension	2	Assumes a decerebrate position
None	1	Doesn't respond; just lies flaccid
Verbal response		
Oriented	5	Is oriented and converses
Confused	4	Is disoriented and confused
Inappropriate words	3	Replies randomly with incorrect words
Incomprehensible	2	Moans or screams
None	1	Doesn't respond
Total score		

Decerebrate and decorticate postures

Decerebrate

The arms are adducted and extended, with the wrists pronated and the fingers flexed. The legs are stiffly extended, with plantar flexion of the feet. Results from damage to the upper brain stem.

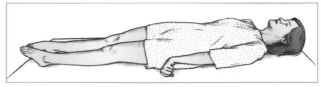

Decorticate

The arms are adducted and flexed, with the wrists and fingers flexed on the chest. The legs are stiffly extended and internally rotated, with plantar flexion of the feet. Results from damage to one or both corticospinal tracts.

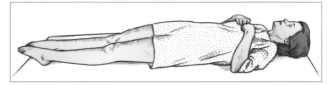

Grading pupil size

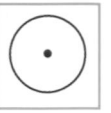
1 mm

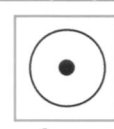
2 mm

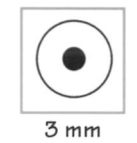
3 mm

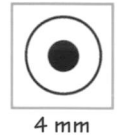
4 mm

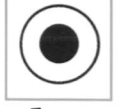
5 mm

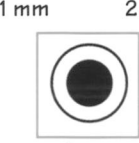
6 mm

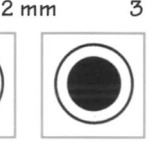
7 mm

8 mm

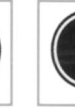
9 mm

Babinski's reflex

Stroking the lateral aspect of the sole of the foot with a thumbnail or another moderately sharp object normally elicits flexion of all toes (a negative Babinski's reflex), as shown below left. In a positive Babinski's reflex, the great toe dorsiflexes and the other toes fan out, as shown below right.

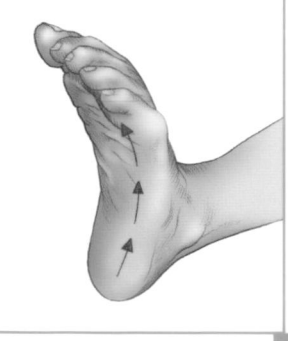

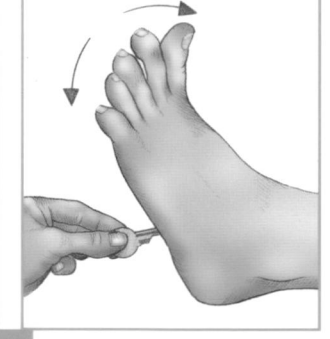

Cranial nerves

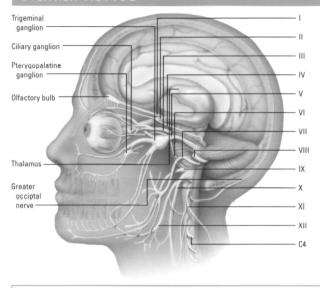

Trigeminal ganglion

Ciliary ganglion

Pterygopalatine ganglion

Olfactory bulb

Thalamus

Greater occipital nerve

I
II
III
IV
V
VI
VII
VIII
IX
X
XI
XII
C4

Cranial nerve function

CN I: Olfactory—Smell
CN II: Optic—Vision
CN III: Oculomotor—Extraocular movement, pupillary constriction, upper eyelid elevation, lens shape change
CN IV: Trochlear—Downward and inward eye movement
CN V: Trigeminal—Chewing, corneal reflex, face and scalp sensations
CN VI: Abducens—Lateral eye movement

CN VII: Facial—Expressions in forehead, eye, and mouth; taste
CN VIII: Acoustic—Hearing and balance
CN IX: Glossopharyngeal—Swallowing, salivating, taste
CN X: Vagus—Swallowing, gag reflex, talking; sensations of throat, larynx, and abdominal viscera
CN XI: Spinal accessory—Shoulder movement, head rotation
CN XII: Hypoglossal—Tongue movement

GI and GU assessment

Inspection

- *GI:* Abdominal symmetry, shape, contour, bumps, bulges, bruises, masses, striae, dilated veins, scars, movement and pulsations, distention, skin tightness, and glistening
- *GU:* Inflammation or discharge from urethral meatus

Palpation

- *GI:* Abdominal size, shape, position; tenderness of major organs; masses and fluid accumulation
- *GU:* Kidneys and bladder

Auscultation

- *GI:* Bowel motility, underlying vessels and organs, bowel sounds (normal, hypoactive, or hyperactive), bruits, venous hum, or friction rub
- *GU:* Renal arteries (with bell in left and right upper abdominal quadrants)

Percussion

- *GI:* Tympany, dullness, size and location of abdominal organs, excessive accumulation of fluid and air (Don't percuss if abdominal aortic aneurysm or transplanted abdominal organ is present.)
- *GU:* Kidneys for tenderness; bladder for position and contents

Abdominal quadrants

Right upper quadrant
- Right lobe of liver
- Gallbladder
- Pylorus
- Duodenum
- Head of the pancreas
- Hepatic flexure of the colon
- Portions of the ascending and transverse colon

Left upper quadrant
- Left lobe of the liver
- Stomach
- Body of the pancreas
- Splenic flexure of the colon
- Portions of the transverse and descending colon

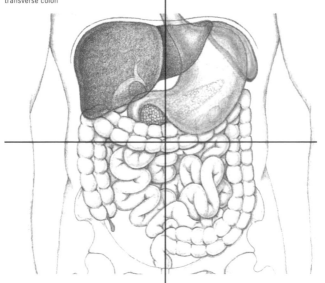

Right lower quadrant
- Cecum and appendix
- Portion of the ascending colon

Left lower quadrant
- Sigmoid colon
- Portion of the descending colon

MUSCULOSKELETAL SYSTEM

Musculoskeletal assessment

Inspection

- No gross deformities.
- Body parts symmetrical.
- Body alignment good.
- No involuntary movements.
- Gait is smooth.
- All muscles and joints have active range of motion with no pain.
- No swelling or inflammation in the joints or muscles.
- Bilateral limb length is equal and muscle mass is symmetrical.

Palpation

- Shape is normal; no swelling or tenderness.
- Bilateral muscle tone, texture, and strength are equal.
- No involuntary contractions or twitching.
- Bilateral pulses are equally strong.

The 5 P's of musculoskeletal injury

To assess a musculoskeletal injury, remember the 5 P's.

Pain

Ask the patient whether he feels pain. If he does, assess the location, severity, and quality of the pain.

Paresthesia

Assess the patient for loss of sensation by touching the injured area with the tip of an open safety pin. Abnormal sensation or loss of sensation indicates neurovascular involvement.

Paralysis

Assess whether the patient can move the affected area. If he can't, he might have nerve or tendon damage.

Pallor

Paleness, discoloration, and coolness on the injured side may indicate neurovascular compromise.

Pulse

Check all pulses distal to the injury site. If a pulse is decreased or absent, blood supply to the area is reduced.

PQRST: The alphabet of pain assessment

Use the PQRST mnemonic device to obtain more information about the patient's pain. Asking the questions below elicits important details about his pain.

Provocative or palliative

- What provokes or worsens your pain?
- What relieves the pain or causes it to subside?

Quality or quantity

- What does the pain feel like? Is it aching, intense, knifelike, burning, or cramping?
- Are you having pain right now? If so, is it more or less severe than usual?
- To what degree does the pain affect your normal activities?
- Do you have other symptoms along with the pain, such as nausea or vomiting?

Region and radiation

- Where is your pain?
- Does the pain radiate to other parts of your body?

Severity

- How severe is your pain? How would you rate it on a 0-to-10 scale, with 0 being no pain and 10 being the worst pain imaginable?
- How would you describe the intensity of your pain at its best? At its worst? Right now?

Timing

- When did your pain begin?
- At what time of day is your pain best? What time is it worst?
- Is the onset sudden or gradual?
- Is the pain constant or intermittent?

Numerical rating scale

A numerical rating scale can help the patient quantify his pain. Have him choose a number from 0 (indicating no pain) to 10 (indicating the worst pain imaginable) to reflect his current pain level. He can either circle the number on the scale itself or verbally state the number that best describes his pain.

No pain 0 1 2 3 4 5 6 7 8 9 10 Pain as bad as it can be

Visual analog scale

To use the visual analog scale, ask the patient to place a mark on the scale to indicate his current level of pain as shown below.

No pain |————————————————| Pain as bad as it can be

Wong-Baker faces pain rating scale

A pediatric patient or an adult patient with language difficulties may not be able to express the pain he's feeling. In such cases, use the pain intensity scale below. Ask the patient to choose the face that best represents the severity of his pain on a scale from 0 to 10.

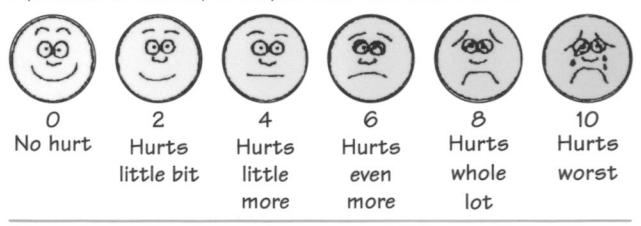

| 0 No hurt | 2 Hurts little bit | 4 Hurts little more | 6 Hurts even more | 8 Hurts whole lot | 10 Hurts worst |

From Wong, D.L., et al. *Wong's Essentials of Pediatric Nursing*, 6th ed. St. Louis: Mosby, Inc., 2001. Reprinted with permission.

Differentiating acute and chronic pain

Acute pain may cause certain physiologic and behavioral changes that you won't observe in a patient with chronic pain.

Type of pain	Physiologic evidence	Behavioral evidence
Acute	• Increased respirations • Increased pulse • Increased blood pressure • Dilated pupils • Diaphoresis	• Restlessness • Distraction • Worry • Distress
Chronic	• Normal respirations, pulse, blood pressure, and pupil size • No diaphoresis	• Reduced or absent physical activity • Despair, depression • Hopelessness

INTEGUMENTARY SYSTEM

Skin assessment

Color

- Bruising
- Discoloration
- Erythema
- Pallor
- Duskiness
- Jaundice
- Cyanosis

Texture

- Thickness
- Mobility
- Roughness
- Smoothness
- Fragility
- Thinness

Turgor

- Returns to regular shape after the skin on the forearm is squeezed: normal; doesn't return to regular shape, returns slowly, or leaves a tented shape: abnormal

Moisture

- Excessive dryness
- Excessive moisture
- Diaphoresis

Temperature

- Generalized or localized coolness or warmth

Lesions

- Vascular changes
- Hemangiomas
- Telangiectases
- Petechiae
- Purpura
- Ecchymosis
- Other lesions

Staging pressure ulcers

You can use pressure ulcer characteristics gained from your assessment to stage the pressure ulcer, as described here. Staging reflects the anatomic depth of exposed tissue. Keep in mind that if the wound contains necrotic tissue, you won't be able to determine the stage until you can see the wound base.

Stage I

• Ulcer presents with a defined area of persistent redness in lightly pigmented skin
• In darker tones, ulcer presents with persistent red, blue, or purple hues

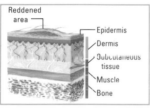

Reddened area — Epidermis
— Dermis
— Subcutaneous tissue
— Muscle
— Bone

Stage II

• Partial-thickness skin loss of epidermis or dermis
• Superficial ulcer
• Presents as abrasion, blister, or shallow crater

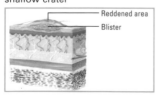

— Reddened area
— Blister

Stage III

• Full-thickness skin loss
• Damage or necrosis of subcutaneous tissue
• May extend down to (but not through) fascia
• Presents as deep crater with or without undermining of adjacent tissue

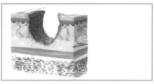

Stage IV

• Full-thickness skin loss
• Extensive destruction, tissue necrosis, or damage to muscle, bone, or support structures
• Possible tunneling and sinus tracts

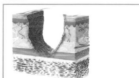

ENDOCRINE SYSTEM

Comparing hypoglycemia, DKA, and HHNS

Hypoglycemia	Diabetic ketoacidosis (DKA)	Hyperosmolar hyperglycemic nonketotic syndrome (HHNS)
Symptom onset		
Rapid (minutes to hours)	Slow (hours to days)	Slow (hours to days), but more gradual than DKA
Signs and symptoms		
Blood pressure Normal or above normal	Subnormal	Subnormal
Breath odor Normal	Fruity, acetone	Normal
GI None	Anorexia, nausea, vomiting, diarrhea, abdominal tenderness and pain	None
Muscle strength Normal or reduced	Extremely weak	Extremely weak
Neurologic status *Initial*—irritability, nervousness, giddiness; hand tremors; difficulty speaking, concentrating, focusing, and coordinating; paresthesia *Late*—hyperreflexia, dilated pupils, coma	*Initial*—dullness, confusion, lethargy; diminished reflexes *Late*—coma	*Initial*—dullness, confusion, lethargy; diminished reflexes *Late*—coma

Comparing hypoglycemia, DKA, and HHNS
(continued)

Hypoglycemia	DKA	HHNS
Signs and symptoms (continued)		
Pulse		
Tachycardic (bradycardic in deep coma)	Mildly tachycardic, weak	Usually rapid
Respirations		
Initial—normal to rapid *Late*—slow	*Initial*—deep, fast *Late*—Kussmaul's	*Initial*—normal *Late*—rapid
Skin and mucous membranes		
Cold, clammy skin; pallor; profuse sweating; normal mucous membranes	Warm, flushed, dry, loose skin; dry, crusty mucous membranes; soft eyeballs	Warm, flushed, dry, extremely loose skin; dry, crusty mucous membranes; soft eyeballs
Temperature		
Commonly subnormal; may be elevated after episode	Hypothermia; possible fever (from dehydration or infection)	Possible fever (from dehydration or infection)
Weight		
Stable	Decreased	Decreased
Other		
Hunger	Thirst	*Initial*—thirst *Late*—possible absence of thirst

(continued)

Comparing hypoglycemia, DKA, and HHNS (continued)

Diagnostic test results	Hypoglycemia	DKA	HHNS
Arterial blood gas levels	Normal or slight respiratory acidosis	Metabolic acidosis with compensatory respiratory alkalosis	Normal or slight metabolic acidosis
Blood glucose level	Below normal (less than 50 mg/dl)	Above normal	Markedly above normal
Hematocrit	Normal	Above normal	Above normal
Serum ketones	Negative	Positive, large	Negative, small
Serum osmolarity	Normal (290 to 310 mOsm/L)	Above normal but usually less than 330 mOsm/L	Markedly above normal (350 to 450 mOsm/L)
Serum potassium level	Normal	Normal or above normal	Normal or above normal
Serum sodium level	Normal	Normal or subnormal	Above normal, normal, or subnormal

Comparing hypoglycemia, DKA, and HHNS
(continued)

Hypoglycemia	DKA	HHNS
Diagnostic test results (continued)		
Urine glucose level		
Normal	Above normal	Markedly above normal
Urine output		
Normal	*Initial*—polyuria *Late*—oliguria	*Initial*—marked polyuria *Late*—oliguria
Treatment		
Glucose, glucagon	Insulin, fluid replacement, electrolyte replacement, antiacidosis therapy (if needed)	Fluid replacement, insulin, electrolyte replacement

Age-related changes

Musculoskeletal system

- Alterations in joint surfaces, ligaments, tendons, and connective tissues
- Decreased bone density
- Decreased number and size of muscle fibers
- Atrophy of muscle tissue; replaced with fibrous tissue

Respiratory system

- Loss of elastic lung recoil
- Increased airway resistance
- Reduced vital capacity
- Decreased chest wall compliance
- Decreased gas exchange

Cardiovascular system

- Increased blood pressure
- Decreased stroke volume
- Decreased cardiac reserve (ability to respond to stress)

Integumentary system

- Decreased subcutaneous adipose tissue
- Decreased elasticity of connective tissue
- Loss of sweat and sebaceous glands

Central nervous system

- Reduced nerve conduction speed
- Decreased rate and magnitude of reflex response
- Decreased sensory activity
- Decreased myoneural transmission
- Decreased muscle contraction speed
- Increased postural sway (contributes to balance problems)

Polypharmacy

Older patients who have multiple disorders sometimes obtain prescriptions from three or four doctors and three or four pharmacies. They might neglect to inform each doctor of the various drugs they're already taking, or a doctor might fail to discontinue previous drugs the patient is taking.

Older patients might also take one or more nonprescription drugs to relieve common complaints, such as stomachache, dizziness, or constipation. Besides the unnecessary expense, this behavior (called *polypharmacy*) increases the risk of adverse drug effects and interactions.

Identifying polypharmacy

Because of your close contact with patients, you're the health care team member who's best able to recognize polypharmacy. Suspect excessive use of drugs if your patient uses:
• several (usually 10 or more) drugs for no logical reason; for example, laxatives that aren't needed
• duplicate drugs, such as sleep sedatives and tranquilizers
• an inappropriate dosage
• contraindicated drugs
• drugs to treat adverse reactions.

Comparing delirium and dementia

This chart highlights distinguishing characteristics of delirium and dementia.

Clinical feature	Delirium	Dementia
Onset	Acute, sudden	Gradual
Course	Short, diurnal fluctuations in symptoms; worse at night, in darkness, and on awakening	Lifelong; symptoms progressive and irreversible
Progression	Abrupt	Slow but uneven
Duration	Hours to less than 1 month; seldom longer	Months to years
Awareness	Reduced	Clear
Alertness	Fluctuates from lethargic to hypervigilant	Generally normal
Attention	Decreased	Generally normal
Orientation	Generally impaired, but reversible	May be impaired as disease progresses
Memory	Recent and immediate impaired	Recent and remote impaired
Thinking	Disorganized, distorted, fragmented; incoherent speech, either slow or accelerated	Difficulty with abstraction; thoughts impoverished; judgment impaired; words difficult to find

Comparing delirium and dementia *(continued)*

Clinical feature	Delirium	Dementia
Perception	Distorted: illusions, delusions, and hallucinations; difficulty distinguishing between reality and misperceptions	Misperceptions usually absent
Speech	Incoherent	Dysphasia as disease progresses; aphasia
Psychomotor behavior	Variable: hypokinetic, hyperkinetic, and mixed	Normal; may have apraxia
Sleep and wake cycle	Altered	Fragmented
Affect	Variable affective anxiety, restlessness, irritability; reversible	Typically superficial, inappropriate, and labile; attempts to conceal deficits in intellect; possible personality changes, aphasia, agnosia; lack of insight
Mental status testing	Distracted from task; numerous errors	Failings highlighted by family; frequent "near miss" answers, struggles with test, great effort to find an appropriate reply; frequent requests for feedback on performance

Elder abuse

Use these guidelines to help evaluate the possibility of abuse of an older adult.

Assessment

- Burns
- Physical or thermal injury on head, face, or scalp
- Bruises and hematomas (unusual location, bruise in the shape of fingerprints, presence of other injuries in different stages of resolution)
- Mental status and neurologic changes from their previous levels
- Fractures, falls, or evidence of physical restraint (such as contractures)
- Ambulation status (poor ambulation or trouble sitting may suggest sexual assault)

Documentation

- Size, shape, and location of injury
- If no new lesions appear during the patient's hospitalization
- If family or caregivers don't visit or show concern
- Abnormal or suspicious behavior of the older person (extremely agitated, fearful, or overly quiet and passive; fearful of caregiver)
- Patient-caregiver interaction

Age-related changes

Age	Developmental markers
1 month	Responds to sound, blinks at bright lights, stares and focuses at faces, lifts head briefly when on stomach
2 months	Smiles in response to caregiver's smile, follows objects with eyes, make noises other than crying
3 months	Holds head steady when upright, laughs and smiles, opens and shuts hands, kicks legs, recognizes faces
4 months	Holds head at 90-degree angle when on stomach, bears weight on both legs, goos and coos when caregiver talks
5 months	Rolls over, reaches out for objects, grasps a rattle or toy, pays attention to small objects held in front of face
6 months	Keeps head level when pulled to sitting position, rolls back and forth, sits momentarily with minimal support, imitates sounds and facial expressions
7 months	Sits without support, makes razzing sounds, feeds self a cracker or finger food, works at getting a toy that's out of reach
8 months	Starts crawling, passes object from one hand to the other, responds to own name, mouths and chews on objects, reaches for spoon when being fed, says "mama" and "dada" to both parents
9 months	Stands while holding on to something, looks for dropped objects, pulls up to standing position from sitting, claps and bangs objects together, may show separation and stranger anxiety

(continued)

Age-related changes (continued)

Age	Developmental markers
10 months	Walks while holding on to furniture, waves good-bye, uses pincer grasp to pick up objects
11 months	Claps hands, understands "no" but doesn't obey it, stands alone momentarily, plays ball and patty-cake
12 months	Babbles, indicates wants with gestures other than crying, exhibits fear of strangers, pulls off socks
13 months	Says two or more words other than "mama" and "dada," stands well, bends over to pick up objects, takes a few steps, walks with help
14 months	Takes a few steps unassisted, empties containers filled with objects, puts objects back in container, eats finger foods
15 months	Toddles well, says up to five words, climbs stairs, likes to look at books, laughs
16 months	Turns pages of a book, gets attached to stuffed animals, walks well, sings, gets upset when frustrated
18 months	Draws a scribble well, runs well, makes a sentence, feeds self with spoon
20 months	Takes off clothes without help, pretends to help toys, imitates caregiver (such as feeding a doll), knows when something is wrong

Age	Developmental markers
2 years	Names at least five or more body parts, uses understandable speech half the time, forms three- or four-word sentences, puts on and takes off clothes alone
3 to 4 years	Uses more than 50 single words, begins to understand cause and effect, socializes, enjoys playing with other children, catches a ball, expresses emotions, can balance on each foot for a second or two, likes to climb obstacles, uses a fork and spoon, may stay dry most nights
5 to 6 years	Can talk in complete sentences, can repeat a sentence, can tell caregiver where they're going, shows signs that separating from parents is easier, ties shoelaces unassisted, skips, jumps rope, stays dry at night almost all of the time, develops very good hand and eye coordination, probably can write and recognize written words
8 to 12 years	Rides bike, reads, counts, ties shoes, skates, uses crayon or pencil well, tends to follow rules, concentrates on playing and learning, forms social relationships
Adolescence	Can think abstractly and form logical conclusions from observations; is preoccupied with appearance, peer expectations, and trying to establish own identity

Recognizing child abuse and neglect

If you suspect a child is being harmed, contact your local child protective services or the police. Contact the Childhelp USA National Child Abuse Hotline (1-800-4-A-CHILD) to find out where and how to file a report.

The following signs may indicate child abuse or neglect.

Children

- Show sudden changes in behavior or school performance
- Haven't received help for physical or medical problems brought to the parent's attention
- Are always watchful, as if preparing for something bad to happen
- Lack adult supervision
- Are overly compliant, passive, or withdrawn
- Come to school or activities early, stay late, and don't want to go home

Parents

- Show little concern for the child
- Deny or blame the child for the child's problems in school or at home
- Request teachers or caregivers use harsh physical discipline if the child misbehaves
- See the child as entirely bad, worthless, or burdensome
- Demand a level of physical or academic performance the child can't achieve
- Look primarily to the child for care, attention, and satisfaction of emotional needs

Parents and children

- Rarely look at each other
- Consider their relationship to be entirely negative
- State that they don't like each other

Signs of child abuse

The following are some signs associated with specific types of child abuse and neglect. These types of abuse are typically found in combination rather than alone.

Physical abuse

- Has unexplained burns, bites, bruises, broken bones, black eyes
- Has fading bruises or marks after absence from school
- Cries when it's time to go home
- Shows fear at approach of adults
- Reports injury by parent or caregiver

Neglect

- Is frequently absent from school
- Begs or steals food or money
- Lacks needed medical or dental care, immunizations, or glasses
- Is consistently dirty and has severe body odor
- Lacks sufficient clothing for the weather

Sexual abuse

- Has difficulty walking or sitting
- Suddenly refuses to change for gym or participate in physical activities
- Reports nightmares or bedwetting
- Demonstrates bizarre, sophisticated, or unusual sexual knowledge or behavior
- Becomes pregnant or contracts a venereal disease when younger than age 14

Emotional maltreatment

- Shows extremes in behavior, such as being overly compliant or demanding, extremely passive, or aggressive
- Is inappropriately adult (e.g., parenting other children) or inappropriately infantile (e.g., frequent rocking or head banging)
- Shows delayed physical or emotional development
- Reports a lack of attachment to the parent
- Has attempted suicide

Psychiatric disorders

Anxiety disorder

Type: Obsessive-compulsive
Symptoms:
• Repetitive thoughts causing stress
• Repetitive behaviors (e.g., hand washing, counting, checking and rechecking door)
• Social impairment due to compulsive behaviors
Treatments:
• Behavioral techniques
• Relaxation techniques
• Medications: Benzodiazepines, MAOIs, SSRIs, TCAs

Mood disorder

Type: Bipolar (manic-depressive)
Symptoms:
• Manic: Elation, euphoria, agitation, hyperexcitability, hyperactivity, rapid thought and speech, decreased sleep
• Depressive: Inertia, social withdrawal, apathy, difficulty concentrating, slowed speech, psychomotor retardation, weight loss, slow gait
Treatments:
• Manic: Lithium, valproic acid
• Depressive: Antidepressants (use cautiously; can trigger manic episode)

Personality disorder

Type: Borderline personality
Symptoms:
• Unstable relationships
• Unstable self-image
• Unstable emotions
• Impulsivity
Treatments:
• Psychotherapy
• Group therapy
• Family therapy
• Medications: Antidepressants, anxiolytics, antimanics, antipsychotics

Psychotic disorder

Type: Schizophrenia
Symptoms:
• Delusions, hallucinations
• Apathy, blunted affect
• Asociality
• Thought disorder
• Bizarre behavior
• Poverty of speech
Treatments:
• Psychosocial treatment and rehabilitation
• Psychotherapy
• Medications: Conventional antipsychotics; atypical antipsychotics (e.g., clozapine)

Psychiatric disorders (continued)

Somatoform disorder

Type: Hypochondriasis
Symptoms:
• Preoccupation with normal body functions
• Sensory, motor, or neurologic symptoms that don't follow a recognizable pattern of organic dysfunction and aren't related to abnormal physical findings

Treatments:
• Psychotherapy
• Cognitive and behavioral therapy
• Medications: Benzodiazepines, SSRIs, TCAs

Suicide's warning signs

• Withdrawal and social isolation
• Signs and symptoms of depression, which may include crying, fatigue, sadness, helplessness, poor concentration, reduced interest in sex and other activities, constipation, and weight loss
• Farewells to friends and family
• Putting affairs in order
• Giving away prized possessions
• Covert suicide messages and death wishes
• Obvious suicide messages, such as: "I'd be better off dead."

Suicide interventions

• Keep communication lines open. Continuity of care and consistency of primary nurses can help.
• Check for dangerous conditions, such as exposed pipes, windows without safety glass, and access to the roof or open balconies.
• Remove belts, sharp objects (such as razors, knives, nail files, and clippers), suspenders, light cords, and glass from the patient's room.
• Make sure an acutely suicidal patient is observed around the clock. Stay alert when he uses a sharp object (as when shaving), takes medications, or uses the bathroom (to prevent hanging or other injury). Assign him a room near the nurses' station and with another patient.

Comprehensive metabolic panel

Test	Conventional units	SI units
Albumin	3.5-5 g/dl	35-50 g/L
Alkaline phosphatase	45-115 units/L	45-115 units/L
ALT	Male: 10-40 units/L	0.17-0.68 μkat/L
	Female: 7-35 units/L	0.12-0.60 μkat/L
AST	12-31 units/L	0.21-0.53 μkat/L
Bilirubin, total	0.2-1 mg/dl	3.5-17 μmol/L
BUN	8-20 mg/dl	2.9-7.5 mmol/L
Calcium	8.2-10.2 mg/dl	2.05-2.54 mmol/L
Carbon dioxide	22-26 mEq/L	22-26 mmol/L
Chloride	100-108 mEq/L	100-108 mmol/L
Creatinine	Male: 0.8-1.2 mg/dl	62-115 μmol/L
	Female: 0.6-0.9 mg/dl	53-97 μmol/L
Glucose	70-100 mg/dl	3.9-6.1 mmol/L
Potassium	3.5-5 mEq/L	3.5-5 mmol/L
Protein, total	6.3-8.3 g/dl	64-83 g/L
Sodium	135-145 mEq/L	135-145 mmol/L

Lipid panel

Test	Conventional units	SI units
Total cholesterol	< 200 mg/dl	< 5.18 mmol/L
HDL cholesterol	≥ 60 mg/dl	≥ 1.55 mmol/L
LDL cholesterol	< 130 mg/dl	< 3.36 mmol/L
VLDL cholesterol	< 130 mg/dl	< 3.4 mmol/L
Triglycerides	< 150 mg/dl	< 1.7 mmol/L

Thyroid panel

Test	Conventional units	SI units
T_3	80-200 ng/dl	1.2-3 nmol/L
T_4, free	0.9-2.3 ng/dl	10-30 nmol/L
T_4, total	5-13.5 mcg/dl	60-165 mmol/L
TSH	0.4-4.2 mIU/L	0.4-4.2 mIU/L

Other chemistry tests

Test	Conventional units	SI units
A/G ratio	3.4-4.8 g/dl	34-38 g/dl
Ammonia	< 50 ng/dl	< 36 µmol/L
Amylase	26-102 units/L	0.4-1.74 µkat/L
Anion gap	8-14 mEq/L	8-14 mmol/L
Bilirubin, direct	< 0.5 mg/dl	< 6.8 µmol/L
Calcitonin	Male: < 16 pg/ml	< 16 ng/L
	Female: < 8 pg/ml	< 8 ng/L
Calcium, ionized	4.65-5.28 mg/dl	1.1-1.25 mmol/L
Cortisol	a.m.: 7-25 mcg/dl	0.2-0.7 µmol/L
	p.m.: 2-14 mcg/dl	0.06-0.39 µmol/L
C-reactive protein	< 0.8 mg/dl	< 8 mg/L
Ferritin	Male: 20-300 ng/ml	20-300 mcg/L
	Female: 20-120 ng/ml	20-120 mcg/L
Folate	1.8-20 ng/ml	4.45-3 nmol/L
GGT	Male: 7-47 units/L	0.12-1.80 µkat/L
	Female: 5-25 units/L	0.08-0.42 µkat/L
Hb_{A1c}	4%-7%	0.04-0.07
Homocysteine	< 12 µmol/L	< 12 µmol/L
Iron	Male: 65-175 mcg/dl	11.6-31.3 µmol/L
	Female: 50-170 mcg/dl	9-30.4 µmol/L
Iron-binding capacity	250-400 mcg/dl	45-72 µmol/L
Lactic acid	0.5-2.2 mEq/L	0.5-2.2 mmol/L
Lipase	10-73 units/L	0.17-1.24 µkat/L
Magnesium	1.3-2.2 mg/dl	0.65-1.05 mmol/L
Osmolality	275-295 mOsm/kg	275-295 mOsm/kg

(continued)

Other chemistry tests (continued)

Test	Conventional units	SI units
Phosphate	2.7-4.5 mg/dl	0.87-1.45 mmol/L
Prealbumin	19-38 mg/dl	190-380 mg/L
Uric acid	Male: 3.4-7 mg/dl	202-416 µmol/L
	Female: 2.3-6 mg/dl	143-357 µmol/L

Tumor markers

Test	Conventional units	SI units
Alpa-fetoprotein	< 40 ng/ml	< 40 mcg/L
CA 15-3	< 30 units/ml	< 30 kU/L
CA 19-9	< 37 units/ml	< 37 kU/L
CA 27-29	$\leq$ 38 units/ml	$\leq$ 38 kU/L
CA 125	< 35 units/ml	< 35 kU/L
Carcinoembryonic antigen	< 2.5-5 ng/ml	< 2.5-5 mcg/L
Human chorionic gonadotropin	< 2 ng/ml	< 2 mcg/L
Neuron-specific enolase	< 12.5 mcg/ml	—
PSA	Age 40-49: $\leq$ 2.5 ng/ml	$\leq$ 2.5 mcg/L
	Age 50-59: $\leq$ 3.5 ng/ml	$\leq$ 3.5 mcg/L
	Age 60-69: $\leq$ 4.5 ng/ml	$\leq$ 4.5 mcg/L
	Age 70+: $\leq$ 6.5 ng/ml	$\leq$ 6.5 mcg/L

Complete blood count with differential

Test	Conventional units	SI units
Hemoglobin	Male: 14-17.4 g/dl	140-174 g/L
	Female: 12-16 g/dl	120-160 g/L
Hematocrit	Male: 42%-52%	0.42-0.52
	Female: 36%-48%	0.36-0.48
RBC	Male: 4.2-5.4 $\times$ 10^6/mm^3	4.2-5.4 $\times$ 10^{12}/L
	Female: 3.6-5 $\times$ 10^6/mm^3	3.6-5 $\times$ 10^{12}/L
MCH	26-34 pg/cell	0.40-0.53 fmol/cell
MCHC	32-36 g/dl	320-360 g/L

Test	Conventional units	SI units
MCV	82-98 mm^3	82-98 fL
WBC	4,000-10,000/cells/mm^3	4-10 × 10^9/L
Bands	0%-5%	0.03-0.08
Basophils	0%-1%	0-0.01
Eosinophils	1%-4%	0.01-0.04
Lymphocytes	25%-40%	0.25-0.40
Monocytes	2%-8%	0.02-0.08
Neutrophils	54%-75%	0.54-0.75
Platelets	140,000-400,000/mm^3	140-400 x 10^9/L

Coagulation studies

Test	Conventional units	SI units
ACT	107 sec ± 13 sec	107 sec ± 13 sec
Bleeding time	3-6 min	3-6 min
D-dimer	< 250 mcg/L	< 1.37 nmol/L
Fibrinogen	200-400 mg/dl	2-4 g/L
INR (target therapeutic)	2.0-3.0	2.0-3.0
Plasminogen	80%-130%	—
PT	10-14 sec	10-14 sec
PTT	21-35 sec	21-35 sec
Thrombin time	10-15 sec	10-15 sec

Other hematology tests

Test	Conventional units	SI units
Erythrocyte sedimentation rate	Male: 0-10 mm/hr	0-10 mm/hr
	Female: 0-20 mm/hr	0-20 mm/hr
Pyruvate kinase	2.8-8.8 units/g Hb	46.7-146.7 μkat/g Hb

Antibiotic peaks and troughs

Test	Conventional units	SI units
Amikacin		
Peak	20-30 mcg/ml	34-52 µmol/L
Trough	1-4 mcg/ml	2-7 µmol/L
Chloramphenicol		
Peak	15-25 mcg/ml	46.4-77 µmol/L
Trough	5-15 mcg/ml	15.5-46.4 µmol/L
Gentamycin		
Peak	4-8 mcg/ml	8.4-16.7 µmol/L
Trough	1-2 mcg/ml	2.1-4.2 µmol/L
Tobramycin		
Peak	4-8 mcg/ml	8.6-17.1 µmol/L
Trough	1-2 mcg/ml	2.1-4.3 µmol/L
Vancomycin		
Peak	25-40 mcg/ml	14-27 µmol/L
Trough	5-10 mcg/ml	3.4-6.8 µmol/L

Urine tests

Test	Conventional units	SI units
Urinalysis		
Appearance	Clear to slightly hazy	—
Color	Straw to dark yellow	—
pH	4.5-8	—
Specific gravity	1.005-1.035	—
Glucose	None	—
Protein	None	—
RBCs	None or rare	—
WBCs	None or rare	—
Osmolality	50-1,400 mOsm/kg	—

Cardiac biomarkers

Protein	Conventional units	SI units	Initial evaluation	Peak	Time to return to normal
Troponin-I	< 0.35 mcg/L	< 0.35 mcg/L	4-6 hr	12 hr	3-10 days
Troponin-T	< 0.1 mcg/L	< 0.1 mcg/L	4-3 hr	12-48 hr	7-10 days
Myoglobin	< 55 rg/ml	< 55 mcg/L	2-4 hr	8-10 hr	24 hr
Hs-CRP	0.020-0.800 mg/dl	0.2-8 mg/L	—	—	Depends on degree of inflammation

Enzyme	Conventional units	SI units	Initial evaluation	Peak	Time to return to normal
CK	Male: 55-170 units/L Female: 30-135 units/L	0.94-2.89 μkat/l 0.51-2.3 μkat/L	—	—	—
CK-MB	< 5%	< 0.05	4-8 hr	12-24 hr	72-96 hr
LD	140-280 units/L	2.34-4.68 μkat/L	2-5 days	—	10 days

Hormone	Conventional units	SI units	Initial evaluation	Peak	Time to return to normal
BNP	< 100 pg/ml	< 100 ng/L	—	—	Depends on severity of heart failure

Crisis values of laboratory tests

Test	Low value	Common causes and effects	High value	Common causes and effects
Ammonia	< 15 mcg SI, < 8.8 µmol/L	Renal failure	> 50 mcg/dl SI, > 29.3 µmol/L	Severe hepatic disease: hepatic coma, Reye's syndrome, GI hemorrhage, heart failure
Calcium, serum	< 6 mg/dl SI, < 1.75 mmol/L	Vitamin D or parathyroid hormone deficiency: tetany, seizures	> 13 mg/dl SI, > 0.3 mmol/L	Hyperparathyroidism: coma
Carbon dioxide and bicarbonate blood	< 10 mEq/L SI, < 10 mmol/L	Complex pattern of metabolic and respiratory factors	> 40 mEq/L SI, > 40 mmol/L	Complex pattern of metabolic and respiratory factors
Creatinine kinase (CK-MB)	—	—	> 5%	Acute MI
Creatinine, serum	—	—	> 4 mg/dl SI, > 353.6 µmol/L	Renal failure: coma
Glucose, blood	< 40 mg/dl SI, < 2.22 mmol/L	Excessive insulin administration, brain damage	> 300 mg/dl SI, > 16.6 mmol/L (with ketonemia and electrolyte imbalance)	Diabetes: diabetic coma

(continued)

Test	Low value	Common causes and effects	High value	Common causes and effects
Hemoglobin	< 8 g/dl SI, < 80 g/L	Hemorrhage or vitamin B₁₂ or iron deficiency; heart failure	> 18 g/dl SI, > 180 g/L	Chronic obstructive pulmonary disease; thrombosis, poly-cythemia vera
International Normalized Ratio	—	—	> 3.0	DIC, uncontrolled oral anticoagulation
Platelet count	< 50 × 10³/mm³ SI, < 50 × 10⁹/L	Bone marrow suppression; hemorrhage	> 500 × 10³/mm³ SI, > 500 × 10⁹/L	Leukemia, reaction to acute bleeding; hemor-rhage
Potassium, serum	< 3 mEq/L SI, < 3 mmol/L	Vomiting and diarrhea, diuretic therapy; car-diotoxicity, arrhythmia, cardiac arrest	> 6 mEq/L SI, > 6 mmol/L	Renal disease, diuretic therapy; cardiotoxicity, arrhythmia
PT	—	—	> 14 sec (> 20 sec for patient on warfarin)	Anticoagulant therapy, anticoagulation factor deficiency; hemor-rhage
PTT	—	—	> 40 sec (> 70 sec for patient on heparin)	Anticoagulation factor deficiency; hemor-rhage

(continued)

Crisis values of laboratory tests (continued)

Test	Low value	Common causes and effects	High value	Common causes and effects
Sodium, serum	< 120 mEq/L SI, < 120 mmol/L	Diuretic therapy; cardiac failure	> 160 mEq/L SI, > 160 mmol/L	Dehydration: vascular collapse
Troponin I	—	—	> 2 mcg/ml SI, > 2 mcg/L	Acute MI
WBC count	< 2,000/cells/mm³ SI, < 2 x 10⁹/L	Bone marrow suppression: infection	> 20,000 cells/mm³ SI, > 20 x 10⁹/L	Leukemia: infection
WBC count, CSF	—	—	> 10 cells/mm³ SI, > 5 x 10⁶/L	Meningitis, encephalitis: infection

Recognizing acid-base disorders

Disorder	ABG findings	Possible causes
Respiratory acidosis (excess CO_2 retention)	• pH < 7.35 • HCO_3^- > 26 mEq/L (if compensating) • $Paco_2$ > 45 mm Hg	• Central nervous system depression from drugs, injury, or disease • Hypoventilation from respiratory, cardiac, musculoskeletal, or neuromuscular disease
Respiratory alkalosis (excess CO_2 loss)	• pH > 7.45 • HCO_3^- < 22 mEq/L (if compensating) • $Paco_2$ < 35 mm Hg	• Hyperventilation due to anxiety, pain, or improper ventilator settings • Respiratory stimulation from drugs, disease, hypoxia, fever, or high room temperature • Gram-negative bacteremia
Metabolic acidosis (HCO_3^- loss or acid retention)	• pH < 7.35 • HCO_3^- < 22 mEq/L • $Paco_2$ < 35 mm Hg (if compensating)	• Depletion of HCO_3^- from renal disease, diarrhea, or small-bowel fistulas • Excessive production of organic acids from hepatic disease, endocrine disorders such as diabetes mellitus, hypoxia, shock, or drug toxicity • Inadequate excretion of acids due to renal disease
Metabolic alkalosis (HCO_3^- retention or acid loss)	• pH > 7.45 • HCO_3^- > 26 mEq/L • $Paco_2$ > 45 mm Hg (if compensating)	• Loss of hydrochloric acid from prolonged vomiting or gastric suctioning • Loss of potassium from increased renal excretion (as in diuretic therapy) or corticosteroid overdose • Excessive alkali ingestion

Dosage calculation formulas and common conversions

Common calculations

$$\text{Body surface area in m}^2 = \sqrt{\frac{\text{height in cm} \times \text{weight in kg}}{3{,}600}}$$

$$\text{mcg/ml} = \text{mg/ml} \times 1{,}000$$

$$\text{ml/minute} = \frac{\text{ml/hour}}{60}$$

$$\text{gtt/minute} = \frac{\text{volume in ml to be infused}}{\text{time in minutes}} \times \text{drip factor in gtt/ml}$$

$$\text{mg/minute} = \frac{\text{mg in bag}}{\text{ml in bag}} \times \text{flow rate} \div 60$$

$$\text{mcg/minute} = \frac{\text{mg in bag}}{\text{ml in bag}} \div 0.06 \times \text{flow rate}$$

$$\text{mcg/kg/minute} = \frac{\text{mcg/ml} \times \text{ml/minute}}{\text{weight in kg}}$$

Common conversions

1 kg = 1,000 g	1 L = 1,000 ml	8 oz = 240 ml
1 g = 1,000 mg	1 ml = 1,000 microliters	1 oz = 30 g
1 mg = 1,000 mcg	1 tsp = 5 ml	1 lb = 454 g
	1 tbs = 15 ml	2.2 lb = 1 kg
1″ = 2.54 cm	2 tbs = 30 ml	

Herb-drug interactions

The use of herbs is becoming more prevalent. It's important to ask the patient if he's using any herbs. Certain herb and drug combinations have potential adverse effects. Monitor the patient closely, and watch for possible reactions.

Herb	Drug	Possible effect
Aloe	Cardiac glycosides, antiarrhythmics	May lead to hypokalemia, which may potentiate cardiac glycosides and antiarrhythmics
	Thiazide diuretics, licorice, and other potassium-wasting drugs	Increases the effects of potassium wasting with thiazide diuretics and other potassium-wasting drugs
	Orally administered drugs	May decrease the absorption of drugs because GI transit time is more rapid
Capsicum	Antiplatelets, anticoagulants	Decreases platelet aggregation and increases fibrinolytic activity, prolonging bleeding time
	Nonsteroidal anti-inflammatory drugs (NSAIDs)	Stimulates GI secretions to help protect against NSAID-induced GI irritation
	Angiotensin-converting enzyme inhibitors	May cause cough
	Theophylline	Increases the absorption of theophylline, possibly leading to higher serum levels or toxicity
	MAOIs	Decreases the effects of MAOIs as a result of increased catecholamine secretion
	CNS depressants (such as opioids, benzodiazepines, or barbiturates)	Increases the sedative effect

(continued)

Herb-drug interactions *(continued)*

Herb	Drug	Possible effect
Capsicum (continued)	Histamine-2 (H₂) blockers, proton pump inhibitors	May decrease effectiveness because of increased acid secretion
Chamomile	Drugs that require GI absorption	May delay drug absorption
	Anticoagulants	May enhance anticoagulant therapy and prolong bleeding time
	Iron	May reduce iron absorption because of the tannic acid content
Echinacea	Immunosuppressants	May counteract immunosuppressant drugs
	Hepatotoxics	May increase hepatotoxicity with drugs that elevate liver enzyme levels
	Warfarin	Increases bleeding time without an increased INR
Evening primrose	Anticonvulsants	Lowers the seizure threshold
Feverfew	Antiplatelets, anticoagulants	May decrease platelet aggregation and increase fibrinolytic activity
	Methysergide	May potentiate methysergide
Garlic	Antiplatelets, anticoagulants	Enhances platelet inhibition, leading to increased anticoagulation
	Insulin, other drugs that cause hypoglycemia	May increase serum insulin levels, causing hypoglycemia, an additive effect with antidiabetics
	Antihypertensives	May increase hypotension
	Antihyperlipidemics	May have additive lipid-lowering properties

Herb	Drug	Possible effect
Ginger	Chemotherapeutic drugs	May reduce nausea associated with chemotherapy
	H_2 blockers, proton pump inhibitors	May decrease effectiveness because of increased acid secretion by ginger
	Antiplatelets, anticoagulants	Inhibits platelet aggregation by antagonizing thromboxane synthase and enhancing prostacyclin, leading to prolonged bleeding time
	Calcium channel blockers	May increase calcium uptake by myocardium, leading to altered drug effects
	Antihypertensives	May antagonize the antihypertensive effect
Ginkgo	Antiplatelets, anticoagulants	May enhance platelet inhibition, leading to increased anticoagulation
	Anticonvulsants	May decrease the effectiveness of anticonvulsants
	Drugs that lower the seizure threshold	May further reduce the seizure threshold
Ginseng	Stimulants	May potentiate the stimulant effects
	Warfarin	May antagonize warfarin, resulting in decreased INR
	Antibiotics	May enhance the effects of some antibiotics (Siberian ginseng)
	Antiplatelets, anticoagulants	Decreases platelet adhesiveness
	Digoxin	May falsely elevate digoxin levels
	MAOIs	Potentiates the action of MAOIs

(continued)

Herb-drug interactions (continued)

Herb	Drug	Possible effect
Ginseng (continued)	Hormones, anabolic steroids	May potentiate the effects of hormone and anabolic steroid therapies (estrogen effects of ginseng may cause vaginal bleeding and breast nodules)
	Alcohol	Increases alcohol clearance, possibly by increasing the activity of alcohol dehydrogenase
	Furosemide	May decrease the diuretic effect of furosemide
	Antipsychotics	May stimulate CNS activity
Glucosamine	Insulin and antidiabetic agents	May cause insulin and oral antidiabetic agents to be less effective
Grapeseed	Warfarin	Increases the effects and the INR as a result of the tocopherol content of grapeseed
Green tea	Warfarin	Decreases effectiveness as a result of the vitamin K content of green tea
Hawthorn berry	Digoxin	Causes an additive positive inotropic effect, with the potential for digoxin toxicity
Kava	CNS stimulants or depressants	May interfere with CNS stimulant therapy
	Benzodiazepines	May result in comalike states
	Alcohol, other CNS depressants	Potentiates the depressant effect of alcohol and other CNS depressants
	Levodopa	Decreases the effectiveness of levodopa
Licorice	Digoxin	Causes hypokalemia, which predisposes the patient to digoxin toxicity

Herb	Drug	Possible effect
Licorice *(continued)*	Hormonal contraceptives	Increases fluid retention and the potential for increased blood pressure as a result of fluid overload
	Corticosteroids	Causes additive and enhanced effects of corticosteroids
	Spironolactone	Decreases the effects of spironolactone
Nettle	Anticonvulsants	May increase sedative adverse effects and the risk of seizure
	Opioids, anxiolytics, hypnotics	May increase sedative adverse effects
	Warfarin	Decreases effectiveness as a result of the vitamin K content of the aerial parts of nettle
	Iron	May reduce iron absorption because of the tannic acid content
St. John's wort	SSRIs, MAOIs, nefazodone, trazodone	Causes additive effects with SSRIs, MAOIs, and other antidepressants, potentially leading to serotonin syndrome, especially when combined with SSRIs
	Indinavir, human immunodeficiency virus protease inhibitors (PIs), nonnucleoside reverse transcriptase inhibitors (NNRTIs)	Induces the cytochrome P-450 metabolic pathway, which may decrease the therapeutic effects of drugs that use this pathway for metabolism (use of St. John's wort and PIs or NNRTIs should be avoided because of the potential for subtherapeutic antiretroviral levels and insufficient virologic response that could lead to resistance or class cross-resistance)
	Opioids, alcohol	Enhances the sedative effects of opioids and alcohol *(continued)*

Herb-drug interactions *(continued)*

Herb	Drug	Possible effect
St. John's wort *(continued)*	Photosensitizing drugs	Increases photosensitivity
	Sympathomimetic amines (such as pseudoephedrine)	Causes additive effects
	Digoxin	May reduce serum digoxin concentrations, decreasing the therapeutic effects
	Reserpine	Antagonizes the effects of reserpine
	Hormonal contraceptives	Increases breakthrough bleeding when taken with hormonal contraceptives; also decreases the effectiveness of the contraceptive
	Theophylline	May decrease serum theophylline levels, making the drug less effective
	Anesthetics	May prolong the effect of anesthetic drugs
	Cyclosporine	Decreases cyclosporine levels to less than therapeutic levels, threatening the rejection of transplanted organs
	Iron	May reduce iron absorption because of the tannic acid content
	Warfarin	May alter the INR; reduces the effectiveness of anticoagulant, requiring increased dosage of the drug

Pharmacokinetics in older adults

Differences in the way older people absorb, distribute, metabolize, and eliminate drugs can alter the effects of medications. The age-related differences are listed below.

Absorption

- Change in quality and quantity of digestive enzymes
- Increased gastric pH
- Decreased number of absorbing cells
- Decreased GI motility
- Decreased intestinal blood flow
- Decreased GI emptying time

Distribution

- Decreased cardiac output and reserve
- Decreased blood flow to target tissues, liver, and kidneys
- Decreased distribution space and area
- Decreased lean body mass
- Increased adipose stores
- Decreased plasma protein (decreases protein-binding drugs)
- Decreased total body water

Metabolism

- Decreased microsomal metabolism of drug
- Decreased hepatic biotransformation

Elimination

- Decreased renal excretion of drug
- Decreased glomerular filtration
- Decreased renal tubular secretion

Drugs causing confusion in older adults

These drug classes can cause confusion in older adults:

- antiarrhythmics
- anticholinergics
- antiemetics
- antihistamines
- antihypertensives
- antiparkinsonian agents
- antipsychotics
- diuretics
- histamine blockers
- opioid analgesics
- sedative-hypnotics
- tranquilizers.

Medications associated with falls

This chart highlights some classes of drugs that are commonly prescribed for older patients and the possible adverse effects of each that may increase a patient's risk of falling.

Drug class	Adverse effects
Alcohol	• Intoxication • Motor incoordination • Agitation • Sedation • Confusion
Antidiabetic drugs	• Acute hypoglycemia
Antihypertensives	• Hypotension
Antipsychotics	• Orthostatic hypotension • Muscle rigidity • Sedation
Benzodiazepines and antihistamines	• Excessive sedation • Confusion • Paradoxical agitation • Loss of balance

Drug class	Adverse effects
Diuretics	• Hypovolemia • Orthostatic hypotension • Electrolyte imbalance
Hypnotics	• Excessive sedation • Ataxia • Poor balance • Confusion • Paradoxical agitation
Opioids	• Hypotension • Sedation • Motor incoordination • Agitation
TCAs	• Orthostatic hypotension

I.M. injection sites

Deltoid

If the volume to be administered is greater than 2 ml, don't use this site.

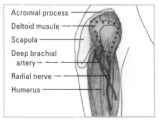

- Acromial process
- Deltoid muscle
- Scapula
- Deep brachial artery
- Radial nerve
- Humerus

Ventrogluteal

This is the preferred injection site for adults and children older than 7 months.

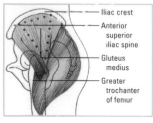

- Iliac crest
- Anterior superior iliac spine
- Gluteus medius
- Greater trochanter of femur

Dorsogluteal

If the site isn't identified properly, damage to the sciatic nerve can occur.

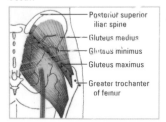

- Posterior superior iliac spine
- Gluteus medius
- Gluteus minimus
- Gluteus maximus
- Greater trochanter of femur

Vastus lateralis

The use of the middle third of this muscle is the preferred site for the neonate.

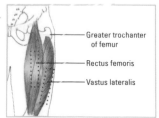

- Greater trochanter of femur
- Rectus femoris
- Vastus lateralis

Z-track injection

1. Place your finger on the skin surface. Pull the skin and subcutaneous layers out of alignment with the underlying muscle. (Move the skin about ½″ [1.3 cm].)

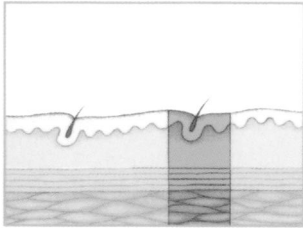

2. Insert the needle at a 90-degree angle where you initially placed your finger.

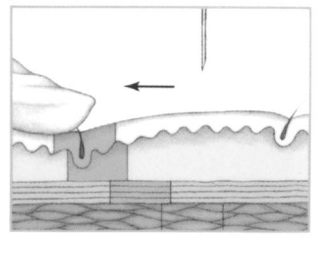

3. Inject the drug and withdraw the needle.

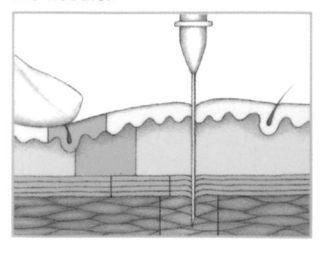

4. Remove your finger from the skin surface, allowing the layers to return to their normal positions.

The needle track (shown by the dotted line) is now broken at the junction of each tissue layer, trapping the drug in the muscle.

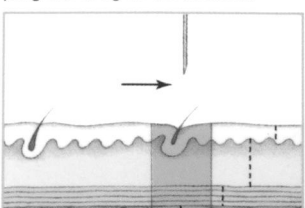

Technique for subQ injections

Before giving the injection, elevate the subcutaneous tissue at the site by grasping it firmly, as shown at right. Insert the needle at a 45- or 90-degree angle to the skin surface, depending on needle length and the amount of subcutaneous tissue at the site.

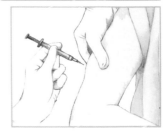

Some medications, such as heparin, should always be injected at a 90-degree angle.

SubQ injection sites

Potential subQ injection sites (as indicated by the dotted areas in the illustration below) include the fat pads on the abdomen, upper hips, upper back, and lateral upper arms and thighs.

Preferred injection sites for insulin are the arms, abdomen, thighs, and buttocks. The preferred injection site for heparin is the lower abdomen fat pad, just below the umbilicus.

For subQ injections administered repeatedly, such as insulin, rotate sites.

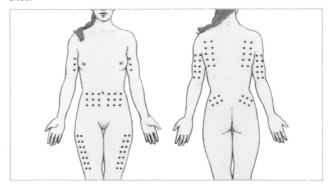

Insulin overview

Insulin type	Onset	Peak (hr)	Usual effective duration (hr)	Usual maximum duration (hr)
Animal				
Regular	0.5-2 hr	3-4	4-6	6-8
NPH	4-6 hr	8-14	16-20	20-24
Human				
Insulin aspart	5-10 min	1-3	3-5	4-6
Insulin lispro	< 15 min	0.5-1.5	2-4	4-6
Regular	0.5-1 hr	2-3	3-6	6-10
NPH	2-4 hr	4-10	10-16	14-18
Lente	3-4 hr	4-12	12-18	16-20
Ultralente	6-10 hr	—	18-20	20-24
Insulin glargine	1 hr	—	24	24

Mixing insulin

When mixing insulin, always draw up clear insulin first, then cloudy.

To mix insulin, follow these steps:
• Wipe the rubber top of the insulin vials with alcohol.
• Gently roll the cloudy insulin between your palms.
• Remove the needle cap.
• Pull out the plunger until the end of the plunger in the barrel aligns with the number of units of cloudy insulin that you need.
• Push the needle through the rubber top of the cloudy insulin bottle.
• Inject air into the bottle.
• Remove the needle.
• Pull out the plunger until the end of the plunger in the barrel

aligns with the units of clear insulin that you need.
• Push the needle through the rubber top of the clear insulin bottle.
• Inject the air into the bottle.
• Without removing the needle, turn the bottle upside down.
• Withdraw the plunger until it aligns with the number of units of clear regular insulin that you need.
• Gently pull the needle out of the bottle.
• Push the needle into the cloudy insulin bottle without injecting the clear insulin into the bottle.
• Withdraw the plunger until you reach your total dosage of insulin in units (clear combined with cloudy).

Insulin infusion pumps

A subQ insulin infusion pump provides continuous, long-term insulin therapy for patients with type 1 diabetes mellitus. Complications include site infection, catheter clogging, and insulin loss from loose reservoir-catheter connections. Insulin pumps work on either an open-loop or a closed-loop system.

Open-loop system

• It's the most common.
• Infuses insulin but can't respond to changes in patient's serum glucose levels.
• Delivers insulin in small (basal) doses every few minutes; large (bolus) doses are set by patient.
• Consists of reservoir-containing insulin syringe, small pump, infusion-rate selector that allows insulin release adjustments, battery, and plastic catheter with attached needle leading from syringe to subQ injection site.
• Needle is held in place with waterproof tape.
• Pump is worn on a belt or in a pocket.
• Infusion line must have clear path to injection site.
• Infusion-rate selector releases about one-half the total daily insulin.
• Patient releases the remainder in bolus doses before meals and snacks.
• Patient must change syringe daily.
• Patient must change needle, catheter, and injection site every other day.

Closed-loop system

• Self-contained; detects and responds to changing serum glucose levels.
• Includes glucose sensor, programmable computer, power supply, pump, and insulin reservoir.
• The computer triggers continuous insulin delivery in appropriate amounts.

Nonneedle catheter system

• Uses tiny plastic catheter inserted into the skin over a needle using a special insertion device.
• The needle is withdrawn, leaving the catheter in place (in the abdomen, thigh, or flank.)
• Catheter is changed every 2 to 3 days.

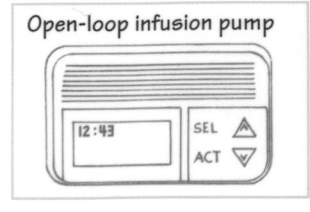

Open-loop infusion pump

Starting an I.V. infusion

Getting ready

- Use the largest vein and the smallest gauge catheter.
- Apply a tourniquet 4" to 6" (10 to 15.5 cm) above the puncture site.
- Leave the tourniquet in place for no more than 3 minutes.
- Lower the patient's arm below the heart and have him pump his fist (not make a fist).
- Try the cephalic and basilic veins first. (They have large lumens and the best blood flow, and are more durable and comfortable.)
- Lightly palpate the vein with the index and middle fingers of your nondominant hand.
- Stretch the skin to anchor the vein.
- Put on gloves and clean the site with a facility-approved antimicrobial solution using a vigorous side-to-side motion.
- If you're using 2% chlorhexidine gluconate swabs, use a vigorous back-and-forth motion, then allow 30 seconds for the solution to dry.
- If you're using 70% isopropyl alcohol or 10% povidone-iodine, use concentric circles, starting in the center and cleaning a diameter 2" to 3" (5 to 7.5 cm).

- The drying time is 30 seconds for 70% isopropyl alcohol and 2 minutes for povidone-iodine.
- Lightly press the skin with the thumb of your nondominant hand about 1½" (3.8 cm) from the intended insertion site.

Inserting the device

- Open the I.V. catheter package and inspect the catheter for flaws or contamination. If any are found, discard it and obtain another catheter.
- Apply traction to the skin and anchor the vein with your nondominant hand, but don't touch the area just beside or directly over the vein.
- Insert the needle bevel up, and advance it until blood appears in the flashback chamber.
- Lower the catheter or needle angle so that it's parallel with the skin and then insert it a little bit more to ensure that the catheter tip is in the vein.
- Verify that blood continues to flow into the flashback chamber.
- If flashback stops and the chamber isn't full, slowly and carefully back out the catheter until flashback returns.

(continued)

Starting an I.V. infusion *(continued)*

• Holding the needle or stylet steady, use your index finger or nondominant hand to gently slide the catheter over the needle and into the vein up to the hub.

• Follow the manufacturer's instructions for catheter advancement and activation of the safety feature.

• Stop immediately if you meet resistance or if the patient complains of severe pain.

• Release the tourniquet and apply digital pressure proximal to the insertion site on the vein to minimize blood backflow.

• Hold the primed extension set; remove the stylet from the catheter hub, activating the safety feature.

• Attach the extension set to the hub of the catheter and flush to verify patency.

• Secure the catheter with tape per your facility's policy.

• Apply a transparent dressing over the site.

• Document which arm was used; anatomic name of vein; catheter gauge, length, and brand; and number of attempts. Quote the patient regarding how the I.V. feels.

Common veins

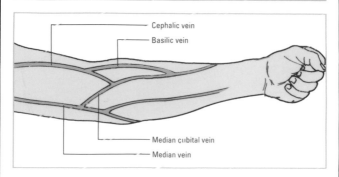

- Cephalic vein
- Basilic vein
- Median cubital vein
- Median vein

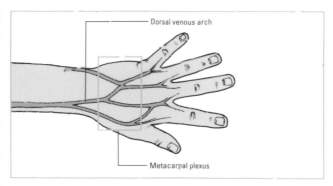

- Dorsal venous arch
- Metacarpal plexus

Local complications of peripheral I.V. lines

Type	Finding	Intervention
Phlebitis	• Tenderness at site • Redness at tip of catheter and along vein	• Remove device. • Apply warm soaks. • Notify doctor.
Infiltration (nonvesicant solution)	• Coolness at site • Skin taut • Slowing of rate	• Remove device. • Apply cold compresses.
Extravasation (vesicant solution)	• Swelling at site • Discomfort (pain, burning) at site • Blanching	• Remove device. • Notify doctor. • Treat site per I.V. solution recommendations.
Catheter dislodgment	• Catheter backed out of vein • Solution inflitrating	• Remove device.
Severed catheter	• Leakage from catheter shaft	• Notify doctor. • If part of catheter enters bloodstream, place tourniquet above I.V. site to prevent progression of broken part.
Hematoma	• Tenderness at site • Bruised area around site	• Remove device. • Apply pressure, cold compresses. • Apply warm soaks.
Venous spasm	• Pain along vein; blanched skin • Flow rate sluggish with clamp open	• Decrease flow rate.

Local complications of peripheral I.V. lines
(continued)

Type	Finding	Intervention
Vasovagal reaction	• Sudden collapse of vein during venipuncture • Sudden pallor, sweating, faintness, dizziness, nausea, and hypotension	• Lower head of bed • Check vital signs. • Have patient take deep breaths.
Thrombosis	• Painful, red, swollen vein • Sluggish or stopped I.V. flow	• Remove device. • Apply warm soaks. • Notify doctor.
Thrombophlebitis	• Severe discomfort at site • Reddened, swollen, hardened vein	• Follow interventions for thrombosis.
Nerve, tendon, or ligament damage	• Extreme pain (like electric shock when nerve is punctured), numbness, and muscle contraction • Delayed effects: paralysis, numbness, and deformity	• Stop procedure. • Notify doctor.

Troubleshooting I.V. pump alarms

A number of electronic devices are available that assist the nurse in controlling the rate and volume of solution infusion. The most common device is an I.V. pump. Safe use of an I.V. requires an understanding of potential device alarms.

Alarm	Possible cause	Intervention
Air in tubing	• Empty I.V. bag	• Spike new I.V. bag and reprime tubing.
	• Hole in I.V. tubing	• Change I.V. tubing.
Low battery power	• Unplugged for extended period of time	• Plug in device.
	• Loss of power to outlet	• Move plug to another outlet.
		• Move plug to emergency outlet.
Downstream occlusion alarm	• Clotted catheter	• Flushing will determine clotting; select new site.
	• I.V. dressing too tight	• Change dressing.
	• Infiltration	• Remove catheter; change site.
	• Kinked tubing	• Locate and remove kink.
	• Filter or extension tubing added	• Stop infusions before adding filters or extensions to tubing and allow pump to establish a new baseline resistance.
	• Addition of a viscous solution	• Allow pump to establish a new baseline pressure.
	• Catheter gauge and tubing length	• Select the smallest catheter that will accept the desired flow rate and the largest vein available.

Central vascular access devices (CVADs) tips and timesavers

- The tip of a CVAD should rest in the superior vena cava. (An exception is a femoral line, which rests in the inferior vena cava.)
- Before giving meds through a CVAD, make sure that an X-ray has verified correct tip placement.
- Document catheter tip placement on flow sheet or med infusion record.
- For PICC catheters, measure external length and compare with previously documented lengths.
- Obtain a blood return from the CVAD before each use.
- When giving meds through a CVAD, use the SASH method for flushing — Saline, Administer the drug (or withdraw blood), Saline, Heparin.
- Refer to your institution's policies and procedures for information on solution volume and frequency of flushing. The established policies and procedures should be based on manufacturer's guidelines.
- Use only a 10-ml or larger syringe to flush a CVAD. The larger the syringe barrel, the lower the pressure. Small-barrel, high-pressure syringes increase the chance of breaking the catheter.
- Flush a CVAD using the positive-pressure technique. Inject the flush, leave your thumb on the syringe plunger, and close the clamp. This helps prevent blood backflow and decreases the chance of catheter occlusion.
- Don't apply ointment at the CVAD insertion site. Use ointment only after catheter removal to occlude the site.

Calculating drip rates

When calculating the flow rate of I.V. solutions, remember that the number of drops required to deliver 1 ml varies with the type of administration set. To calculate the drip rate, you must know the calibration of the drip rate for each specific manufacturer's product. As a quick guide, refer to the chart below. Use this formula to calculate specific drip rates:

$$\frac{\text{volume of infusion (in ml)}}{\text{time of infusion (in minutes)}} \times \text{drip factor (in drops/ml)} = \text{drops/minute}$$

	Ordered volume					
	500 ml/24 hr or 21 ml/hr	1,000 ml/24 hr or 42 ml/hr	1,000 ml/20 hr or 50 ml/hr	1,000 ml/10 hr or 100 ml/hr	1,000 ml/8 hr or 125 ml/hr	1,000 ml/6 hr or 167 ml/hr
Drops/ml	**Drops/minute to infuse**					
Macrodrip						
10	4	7	8	17	21	28
15	5	11	13	25	31	42
20	7	14	17	33	42	56
Microdrip						
60	21	42	50	100	125	167

Tips for high-risk drips

PCA, heparin, and insulin infusions can be especially dangerous if administered incorrectly. If possible, have another nurse independently check the doctor's order, your calculations, and the pump settings for these drugs before starting them.

PCA

Be sure to note the:
• strength of the drug solution in the syringe
• number of drug administrations during assessment period
• basal dose patient received, if any
• amount of solution received (number of injections × volume of injections + basal doses)
• total amount of drug received (amount of solution × solution strength).

Heparin

Be sure to:
• determine the solution's concentration (Divide the units of drug added by the amount of the solution in milliliters.)
• state as a fraction: the desired dose over the unknown flow rate
• cross-multiply to find the flow rate.

Insulin

Be sure to:
• remember that regular insulin is the only type given by I.V. route
• always use an infusion pump
• use concentrations of 1 unit/ml.

Vascular access ports

A vascular access port (VAP) is used to deliver intermittent infusions of medication, chemotherapy, and blood products. Because the device is completely covered by the patient's skin, the risk of extrinsic contamination is reduced. The device doesn't alter the body image and requires less routine catheter care.

The VAP consists of a catheter connected to a small reservoir. A septum designed to withstand multiple punctures seals the reservoir.

Accessing VAP

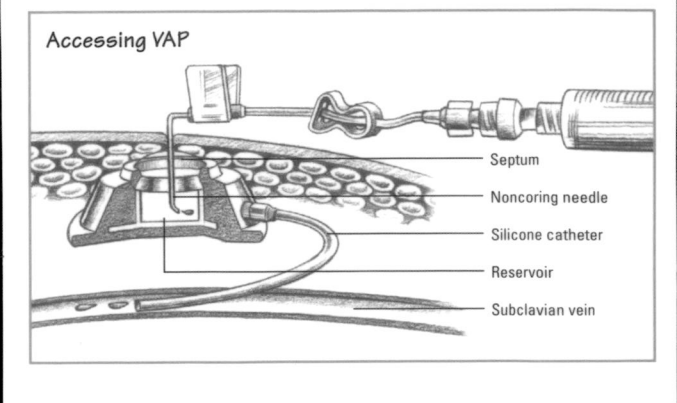

- Septum
- Noncoring needle
- Silicone catheter
- Reservoir
- Subclavian vein

INFUSION RATES

Epinephrine and isoproterenol infusion rates

Epinephrine

Mix 1 mg in 250 ml (4 mcg/ml).

Dose (mcg/min)	Infusion rate (ml/hr)
1	15
2	30
3	45
4	60
5	75
6	90
7	105
8	120
9	135
10	150
15	225
20	300
25	375
30	450
35	525
40	600

Isoproterenol

Mix 1 mg in 250 ml (4 mcg/ml).

Dose (mcg/min)	Infusion rate (ml/hr)
0.5	8
1	15
2	30
3	45
4	60
5	75
6	90
7	105
8	120
9	135
10	150
15	225
20	300
25	375
30	450

Nitroglycerin infusion rates

Determine the infusion rate in ml/hr using the ordered dose and the concentration of the drug solution.

Dose (mcg/min)	25 mg/250 ml (100 mcg/ml)	50 mg/250 ml (200 mcg/ml)	100 mg/250 ml (400 mcg/ml)
5	3	2	1
10	6	3	2
20	12	6	3
30	18	9	5
40	24	12	6
50	30	15	8
60	36	18	9
70	42	21	10
80	48	24	12
90	54	27	14
100	60	30	15
150	90	45	23
200	120	60	30

Dobutamine infusion rates

Mix 250 mg in 250 ml of D$_5$W (1,000 mcg/ml). Determine the infusion rate in ml/hr using the ordered dose and the patient's weight in pounds or kilograms.

Dose (mcg/ kg/min)		Patient's weight												
lb 88	99	110	121	132	143	154	165	176	187	198	209	220	231	242
kg 40	45	50	55	60	65	70	75	80	85	90	95	100	105	110
2.5	6	7	8	8	9	10	11	11	12	13	14	14	15	16	17
5	12	14	15	17	18	20	21	23	24	26	27	29	30	32	33
7.5	18	20	23	25	27	29	32	34	36	38	41	43	45	47	50
10	24	27	30	33	36	39	42	45	48	51	54	57	60	63	66
12.5	30	34	38	41	45	49	53	56	60	64	68	71	75	79	83
15	36	41	45	50	54	59	63	68	72	77	81	86	90	95	99
20	48	54	60	66	72	78	84	90	96	102	108	114	120	126	132
25	60	68	75	83	90	98	105	113	120	128	135	143	150	158	165
30	72	81	90	99	108	117	126	135	144	153	162	171	180	189	198
35	84	95	105	116	126	137	147	158	168	179	189	200	210	221	231
40	96	108	120	132	144	156	168	180	192	204	216	228	240	252	264

Dopamine infusion rates

Mix 400 mg in 250 ml of D_5W (1,600 mcg/ml). Determine the infusion rate in ml/hr using the ordered dose and the patient's weight in pounds or kilograms.

Dose (mcg/kg/min)	lb 88 kg 40	99 45	110 50	121 55	132 60	143 65	154 70	165 75	176 80	187 85	198 90	209 95	220 100	231 105
2.5	4	4	5	5	6	6	7	7	8	8	8	9	9	10
5	8	8	9	10	11	12	13	14	15	16	17	18	19	20
7.5	11	13	14	15	17	18	20	21	23	24	25	27	28	30
10	15	17	19	21	23	24	26	28	30	32	34	36	38	39
12.5	19	21	23	26	28	30	33	35	38	40	42	45	47	49
15	23	25	28	31	34	37	39	42	45	48	51	53	56	59
20	30	34	38	41	45	49	53	56	60	64	68	71	75	79
25	38	42	47	52	56	61	66	70	75	80	84	89	94	98
30	45	53	56	62	67	73	79	84	90	96	101	107	113	118
35	53	59	66	72	79	85	92	98	105	112	118	125	131	138
40	60	68	75	83	90	98	105	113	120	128	135	143	150	158
45	68	76	84	93	101	110	118	127	135	143	152	160	169	177
50	75	84	94	103	113	122	131	141	150	159	169	178	188	197

Patient's weight

Nitroprusside infusion rates

Mix 50 mg in 250 ml of D_5W (200 mcg/ml). Determine the infusion rate in ml/hr using the ordered dose and the patient's weight in pounds or kilograms.

Dose (mcg/kg/min)	Patient's weight														
lb	88	99	110	121	132	143	154	165	176	187	198	209	220	231	242
kg	40	45	50	55	60	65	70	75	80	85	90	95	100	105	110
0.3	4	4	5	5	5	6	6	7	7	8	8	9	9	9	10
0.5	6	7	8	8	9	10	11	11	12	13	14	14	15	16	17
1	12	14	15	17	18	20	21	23	24	26	27	29	30	32	33
1.5	18	20	23	25	27	29	32	34	36	38	41	43	45	47	50
2	24	27	30	33	36	39	42	45	48	51	54	57	60	63	66
3	36	41	45	50	54	59	63	68	72	77	81	86	90	95	99
4	48	54	60	66	72	78	84	90	96	102	108	114	120	126	132
5	60	68	75	83	90	98	105	113	120	128	135	143	150	158	165
6	72	81	90	99	108	117	126	135	144	153	162	171	180	189	198
7	84	95	105	116	126	137	147	158	168	179	189	200	210	221	231
8	96	108	120	132	144	156	168	180	192	204	216	228	240	252	264
9	108	122	135	149	162	176	189	203	216	230	243	257	270	284	297
10	120	135	150	165	180	195	210	225	240	255	270	285	300	315	330

Notes

Meds/IV

CPR

Before beginning basic life support, CPR, or rescue breathing, activate the appropriate code team.

Adult or adolescent

Check for unresponsiveness	Gently shake and shout, "Are you okay?"
Call for help/call 911	Immediately call 911 for help. If a second rescuer is available, send him to get help or an AED and initiate CPR if indicated. If asphyxial arrest is likely, perform 5 cycles (about 2 min) of CPR before activating EMS.
Position patient	Place patient in supine position on hard, flat surface.
Open airway	Use head-tilt, chin-lift maneuver unless contraindicated by trauma.
If you suspect trauma	Open airway using jaw-thrust method if trauma is suspected.
Check for adequate breathing	Look, listen, and feel for 10 sec.
Perform ventilations	Do two breaths initially that make the chest rise at 1 second/breath; then one every 5 to 6 sec.
If chest doesn't rise	Reposition and reattempt ventilation. Several attempts may be necessary
Check pulse	Palpate the carotid for no more than 10 sec.
Start compressions	
Placement	Place both hands, one atop the other, on lower half of sternum between the nipples, with elbows locked; use straight up-and-down motion without losing contact with chest.
Depth	One-third depth of chest or 1½" to 2"
Rate	100/min
Comp-to-vent ratio	30:2 (if intubated, continuous chest compressions at a rate of 100/min without pauses for ventilation; ventilation at 8 to 10 breaths/min)
Check pulse	Check after 2 min of CPR and as appropriate thereafter. Minimize interruptions in chest compressions.
Use AED	Apply as soon as available and follow prompts. Provide 2 min of CPR after first shock is delivered before activating AED to reanalyze rhythm and attempt another shock.

CPR

Child (1 year to onset of adolescence or puberty)

Check for unresponsiveness	Gently shake and shout, "Are you okay?"
Call for help/call 911	Call after 2 min of CPR. Call immediately for witnessed collapse.
Position patient	Place patient in a supine position on a hard, flat surface.
Open airway	Use head-tilt, chin-lift maneuver unless contraindicated by trauma.
If you suspect trauma	Open airway using jaw-thrust method if trauma is suspected.
Check breathing	Look, listen, and feel for 10 sec.
Perform ventilations	Do two breaths initially that make the chest rise at 1 sec/breath; then one every 3 to 5 sec.
If chest doesn't rise	Reposition and reattempt ventilation. Several attempts may be necessary.
Check pulse	Palpate the carotid or femoral for no more than 10 sec.
Start compressions Placement	Place heel of one hand or place both hands, one atop the other, with elbows locked, on lower half of sternum between the nipples.
Depth	⅓ to ½ depth of the chest
Rate	100/min
Comp:Vent ratio	30:2 (if intubated, continuous chest compressions at a rate of 100/min without pauses for ventilation; ventilation at 8 to 10 breaths/min)
Check pulse	Check after 2 min of CPR and as appropriate thereafter. Minimize interruptions in chest compressions.
AED	Use as soon as available and follow prompts. Use child pads and child system for child age 1 to 8 years. Provide 2 min of CPR after first shock is delivered before activating AED to reanalyze rhythm and attempt another shock.

CPR

Infant (0 to 1 year)

Check for unresponsiveness	Gently shake and flick bottom of foot and call out name.
Call for help/call 911	Call after 2 minutes of CPR; call immediately for witnessed collapse.
Position patient	Place patient in a supine position on a hard, flat surface.
Open airway	Use head-tilt, chin-lift maneuver unless contraindicated by trauma. Don't hyperextend the infant's neck.
If you suspect trauma	Open airway using jaw-thrust method if trauma is suspected.
Check breathing	Look, listen, and feel for 10 seconds.
Perform ventilations	Do two breaths at 1 second/breath initially; then one every 3 to 5 seconds.
If chest doesn't rise	Reposition and reattempt ventilation. Several attempts may be necessary.
Check pulse	Palpate brachial or femoral pulse for no more than 10 seconds.
Start compressions	
Placement	Place two fingers 1 fingerwidth below nipples.
Depth	⅓ to ½ depth of the chest
Rate	100/minute
Comp:Vent ratio	30:2 (If intubated, continuous chest compression at a rate of 100/min. without pauses for ventilation; ventilation at 8 to 10 breaths/min.)
Check pulse	Check after 2 minutes of CPR and as appropriate thereafter. Minimize interruptions in chest compressions.

Choking

Adult or child (older than 1 year)

Symptoms
- Grabbing the throat with the hand
- Inability to speak
- Weak, ineffective coughing
- High-pitched sounds while inhaling

Interventions

1. Shout, "Are you choking? Can you speak?" Assess for airway obstruction. Don't intervene if the person is coughing forcefully and able to speak; a strong cough can dislodge the object.

2. Stand behind the person and wrap your arms around the person's waist (if pregnant or obese, wrap arms around chest).

3. Make a fist with one hand; place the thumbside of your fist just above the person's navel and well below the sternum.

4. Grasp your fist with your other hand.

5. Use quick, upward and inward thrusts with your fist (perform chest thrusts for pregnant or obese victims).

6. Continue thrusts until the object is dislodged or the victim loses consciousness. If the latter occurs, activate the emergency response number and provide CPR. Each time you open the airway to deliver rescue breaths, look in the mouth and remove any object you see. Never perform a blind finger-sweep.

Choking

Infant (younger than 1 year)

Symptoms

- Inability to cry or make significant sound
- Weak, ineffective coughing
- Soft or high-pitched sounds while inhaling
- Bluish skin color

Interventions

1. Assess that airway is obstructed. *Don't* perform the next two steps if infant is coughing forcefully or has a strong cry.
2. Lay infant face down along your forearm. Hold infant's chest in your hand and his jaw with your fingers. Point the infant's head downward, lower than the body. Use your thigh or lap for support.
3. Give five quick, forceful blows between the infant's shoulder blades using the heel of your free hand.

After five blows

1. Turn the infant face up.
2. Place two fingers on the middle of infant's sternum just below the nipples.
3. Give five quick thrusts down, compressing the chest at ⅓ to ½ the depth of the chest or ½" to 1" (2 to 2.5 cm).
4. Continue five back blows and five chest thrusts until the object is dislodged or the infant loses consciousness. If the latter occurs, perform CPR. Each time you open the airway to deliver rescue breaths, look in the mouth and remove any object you see. Never perform a blind finger-sweep.

Pulseless arrest algorithm

1 Initiate BLS.

2 Check rhythm. *Shockable rhythm?*

- **3 YES** — VF/VT
- **9 NO** — Asystole/PEA

VF/VT path

4 Give 1 shock (biphasic: 120 to 20 joules; monophasic: 360 joules).
- Immediately resume CPR.

5 Give 5 cycles of CPR*
Check rhythm. *Shockable rhythm?*
- **YES**

6
- Continue CPR while charging defibrillator.
- Give 1 shock (biphasic: same as first shock or higher dose; monophasic: 360 joules).
- Immediately resume CPR.
- Epinephrine 1 mg I.V. or I.O. Repeat every 3 to 5 min OR give 1 dose of vasopressin 40 units I.V. or I.O. to replace first or second dose of epinephrine.

7 Give 5 cycles of CPR*
Check rhythm. *Shockable rhythm?*
- **YES**
- **NO** — go to box 10.

8
- Continue CPR while charging defibrillator.
- Give 1 shock (biphasic: same as first shock or higher dose; monophasic: 360 joules).
- Immediately resume CPR.
- Consider antiarrhythmics; give during CPR.
- Consider magnesium, loading dose.
- After 5 cycles of CPR*, go to box 5.

Asystole/PEA path

10
- Immediately resume CPR for 5 cycles.
- Give epinephrine 1 mg I.V. or I.O. Repeat every 3 to 5 min OR give 1 dose of vasopressin 40 units I.V. or I.O. to replace first or second dose of epinephrine.
- Consider atropine 1 mg I.V. or I.O. for asystole or slow PEA rate. Repeat every 3 to 5 min (up to 3 doses).

11 Give 5 cycles of CPR*
Check rhythm. *Shockable rhythm?*
- **13 YES** — Go to box 4.
- **12 NO**

12
- If asystole, go to box 10.
- If electrical activity, check pulse. If no pulse, go to box 10.
- If pulse present, begin postresuscitation care.

---

* After an advanced airway is placed, give continuous chest compressions without pauses for breaths.

Rapid sequence intubation

Standard algorithm for adults

Preparation (< 10 min)

Pre-oxygenation (3 to 5 min or eight full vital capacity breaths of 100% oxygen)

Premedicate
a. Sedate (administer premedication—usually fentanyl, atropine [for children], lidocaine, etomidate, ketamine, midazolam, or thiopental—then wait 3 min after drug administration)
b. Paralyze (usually succinylcholine, rocuronium, vecuronium, atracurium, or pancuronium)
c. Assess for apnea and jaw relaxation

Protect airway
Perform cricoid pressure (Sellick maneuver) as soon as patient becomes unconscious and then wait 30 seconds

Intubate (each attempt < 20 seconds; max three attempts)
• If more than 1 attempt needed, ventilate patient for 30 to 60 seconds with bag mask between attempts.
• After intubation, inflate balloon cuff.
• If patient becomes bradycardic during intubation, give atropine 0.5 mg I.V. push.

Verify tube placement (by clinical signs, end-tidal carbon dioxide using a capnometer, or esophageal device detector and by reconfirming that the ET tube actually passes between the cords by repeating direct laryngoscopy)

Post-tube management
• Secure ET tube.
• Set ventilator to appropriate settings.
• Continue administering sedative and muscle relaxant p.r.n.
• Obtain chest X-ray stat.
• Recheck vital signs and pulse oximetry.
• Perform continuous end tidal capnometry (to detect accidental extubation).

Analyzing CO_2 levels

Disposable end-tidal carbon dioxide ($ETco_2$) detectors are commonly used to confirm ET tube placement. The meaning of color changes within the detector dome differ depending on which detector you use. Here's a description of what color changes mean in the Easy Cap detector:

• The rim of the Easy Cap is divided into four segments (clockwise from the top): CHECK, A, B, and C. The CHECK segment is solid purple, signifying the absence of CO_2.

• The numbers in the other sections range from 0.03 to 5, indicating the percentage of exhaled CO_2. The color should fluctuate during ventilation from purple (section A) during inspiration to yellow (section C) at the end of expiration. This indicates that $ETco_2$ levels are adequate (above 2%).

• An end-expiratory color change from C to the B range may be the first sign of hemodynamic instability.

• During CPR, an end-expiratory color change from the A or B range to the C range may mean the return of spontaneous ventilation.

• During prolonged cardiac arrest, inadequate pulmonary perfusion leads to inadequate gas exchange. The patient exhales little or no CO_2, so the color stays in the purple range even with proper intubation. Ineffective CPR also leads to inadequate pulmonary perfusion.

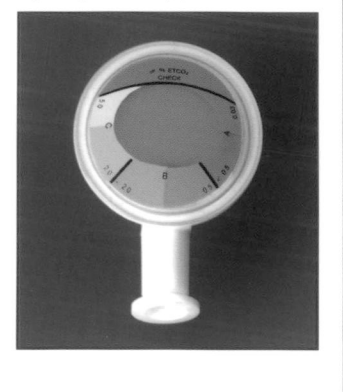

Oxygen therapy

Nasal cannula
- Flow rate of 1 to 6 L/min delivers 24% to 40% FIO_2.
- Headache may occur if flow rate greater than 6 L/minute.

Simple mask*
- Flow rate of 5 to 8 L/min delivers 40% to 60% FIO_2.
- Minimum of 5 L/min needed to flush carbon dioxide from mask and prevent rebreathing it.

Partial rebreather mask*
- Flow rate of 10 L/min delivers 40% to 60% FIO_2.
- Monitor reservoir bag collapse; marked or complete deflation can lead to carbon dioxide accumulation in mask (check oxygen flow).

Nonrebreather mask*
- Flow rate of 6 to 8 L/min delivers 60% to 80% FIO_2.
- Check that one-way valves are secure and functioning.
- Marked or complete deflation of reservoir bag can lead to carbon dioxide accumulation in mask (check oxygen flow).

Venturi mask*
- Flow rate of 4 to 10 L/min delivers 24% to 55% FIO_2.
- Make sure Venturi valve is set for desired FIO_2.

Continuous positive airway pressure (CPAP) mask*
- Variable oxygen concentration.
- Place one strap behind head and other strap over head for snug fit.

Transtracheal oxygen
- Variable oxygen concentration.
- Monitor for irritation, coughing, pain, and respiratory distress.

Aerosols
- Variable; high-humidity oxygen.
- Can be heated or cooled.
- Delivered by a jet nebulizer.

* Mask must fit snugly.

Mechanical ventilation glossary

Assist-control mode: Ventilator delivers a preset rate. Patient can initiate additional breaths, triggering the ventilator to deliver the preset tidal volume at positive pressure.

Continuous positive airway pressure (CPAP): Ventilator delivers positive pressure to the airway throughout the respiratory cycle. Patient must be able to breathe spontaneously.

Control mode: Ventilator delivers a preset tidal volume at a fixed rate whether or not patient is breathing spontaneously.

Fraction of inspired oxygen (FIO$_2$): Amount of oxygen delivered to patient by the ventilator.

Inspiratory flow rate (IFR): Denotes the tidal volume delivered within a certain time. Ranges from 20 to 120 L/min.

Minute ventilation or minute volume (V$_E$): The product obtained by multiplying respiratory rate and tidal volume.

Peak inspiratory pressure (PIP): Amount of pressure required to deliver a preset tidal volume.

Positive end-expiratory pressure (PEEP): Ventilation is triggered to apply positive pressure at the end of each expiration. Helps to inflate and keep open collapsed alveoli.

Respiratory rate: Number of breaths per minute delivered by the ventilator.

Sensitivity setting: Amount of effort patient exerts to trigger the inspiratory cycle.

Sigh volume: Ventilator-delivered breath 1½ times as large as patient's tidal volume.

Synchronized intermittent mandatory ventilation (SIMV): Ventilator delivers a preset number of breaths at a specific tidal volume. Patient may supplement mechanical ventilations with his own breaths.

Tidal volume (V$_T$): Volume of air delivered to patient with each cycle, usually 12 to 15 cc/kg.

Troubleshooting ventilator alarms

Signal	Possible cause	Interventions
Low-pressure alarm	• Tube disconnection	• Reconnect tube to ventilator.
	• ET tube displaced	• Check tube placement; reposition, if needed. If extubation or displacement has occurred, ventilate patient manually. Call doctor immediately.
	• Leaking tidal volume from low cuff pressure	• Listen for whooshing sound around tube, indicating an air leak. If you hear one, check cuff pressure. If you can't maintain pressure, call doctor.
	• Ventilator malfunction	• Disconnect patient from ventilator and ventilate manually, if necessary. Obtain another ventilator.
	• Leak in ventilator circuitry	• Make sure all connections are intact. Check for holes or leaks in tubing. Check humidification jar and replace if cracked.
High-pressure alarm	• Increased airway pressure or decreased lung compliance	• Auscultate lungs for evidence of increasing lung consolidation, barotrauma, or wheezing. Call doctor if indicated.
	• Patient biting on oral ET tube	• Insert bite block if needed.
	• Secretions in airway	• Suction patient or have him cough.
	• Condensate in larger-bore tubing	• Check tubing for condensate and remove any fluid.
	• Intubation of right main stem bronchus	• Check tube position. If it has slipped, call doctor.
	• Patient coughing, gagging, or attempting to talk	• If patient fights the ventilator, doctor may order sedative or neuromuscular blocking agent.
	• Chest wall resistance	• Reposition patient to improve chest expansion. If repositioning doesn't help, administer prescribed analgesics.
	• Failure of high-pressure relief valve	• Replace faulty equipment.
	• Bronchospasm	• Assess for cause. Notify doctor.

Complications of mechanical ventilation and intubation

Mechanical ventilation

- Tension pneumothorax
- Decreased cardiac output
- Infection
- Volutrauma
- Organ impairment (renal, GI, CNS)

Intubation

- Trauma to teeth, lips, tongue
- Vocal cord injury
- Erosion of tracheal wall
- Ischemic pressure necrosis

Interventions for respiratory distress in mechanically ventilated patients

- Disconnect ventilator from ET or trach tube and manually ventilate with Ambu bag at 100% oxygen.
- Check ventilator for problems. Alert respiratory therapy team.
- Assess ET or trach tube for air leak, and check cuff pressure. Notify doctor if air leak isn't corrected.
- Suction ET or trach tube to clear secretions. Continue to ventilate manually.
- If ET tube is dislodged, remove tube and manually ventilate. Notify doctor immediately.
- If trach tube is out, use sterile tracheal dilator to keep stoma open until new tube can be inserted. Notify doctor immediately.

Closed tracheal suctioning

Closed tracheal suctioning permits the patient to remain connected to the ventilator during suctioning. Follow these steps:

1. Remove closed suction system from wrapping. Attach the control valve to connecting tubing.

2. Depress thumb section control valve. Keep it depressed and set suction pressure to desired level.

3. Connect T-piece to ventilator breathing circuit with irrigation port closed.

4. Connect T-piece to ET or trach tube (as shown below).

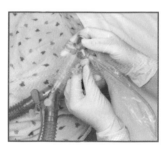

5. With one hand keeping T-piece parallel to patient's chin, use thumb and index finger of other hand to advance catheter through tube and into patient's tracheobronchial tree (as shown below).

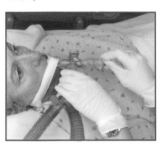

6. If needed, retract catheter sleeve as you advance catheter.

7. Continue to hold T-piece and control valve. Apply intermittent suction and withdraw catheter until it reaches its fully extended length in sleeve. Repeat as needed.

8. When finished, flush catheter by maintaining suction while slowly introducing normal saline solution or sterile water into irrigation port.

9. Place thumb control valve in off position.

10. Dispose of and replace suction equipment according to your facility's policy.

Chest drainage

One-piece disposable plastic drainage systems such as Pleur-Evac contain three chambers:

• The drainage chamber has three calibrated columns that display the amount of drainage collected.
• The water-seal chamber allows air and fluid to escape from the pleural cavity but doesn't allow air to reenter.
• The suction-control chamber is filled with water to achieve various suction levels.
• Rubber diaphragms are provided at the rear of the device to change the water level or remove samples of drainage.
• A positive-pressure relief valve vents excess pressure into the atmosphere, preventing pressure buildup.

Pleur-Evac

Positive-pressure relief valve

To patient

To suction

Suction-control chamber

Water-seal chamber

Drainage chamber

Blood products

Blood component	Indications
Packed RBCs Same RBC mass as whole blood but with 80% of the plasma removed *Volume:* 250 ml	• Inadequate circulating red cell mass • Symptomatic deficiency of oxygen-carrying capacity • Symptomatic chronic anemia • Sickle cell disease (red cell exchange)
Platelets Platelet sediment from RBCs or plasma *Volume:* 35 to 50 ml/unit	• Bleeding due to critically decreased circulating or functionally abnormal platelets • Prevention of bleeding due to thrombocytopenia
Fresh frozen plasma (FFP) Uncoagulated plasma separated from RBCs and rich in coagulation factors V, VIII, and IX *Volume:* 180 to 300 ml	• Coagulation factor deficiency • Warfarin reversal • Thrombotic thrombocytopenic purpura
Albumin 5% (buffered saline); albumin 25% (salt poor) A small plasma protein prepared by fractionating pooled plasma *Volume:* 5% = 12.5 g/250 ml; 25% = 12.5 g/50 ml	• Volume loss because of shock from burns, trauma, surgery, or infections • Hypoproteinemia
Cryoprecipitate Insoluble portion of plasma recovered from FFP *Volume:* approximately 30 ml (freeze-dried)	• Bleeding associated with factor XIII and fibrogen deficiencies

Transfusion reactions

Reaction and causes	Signs and symptoms
Allergic • Allergen in donor blood • Donor blood hypersensitive to certain drugs	Anaphylaxis (chills, facial swelling, laryngeal edema, pruritus, urticaria, wheezing), fever, nausea, and vomiting
Bacterial contamination • Organisms that can survive cold, such as _Pseudomonas_ and _Staphylococcus_	Chills, fever, vomiting, abdominal cramping, diarrhea, shock, signs of renal failure
Febrile • Bacterial lipopolysaccharides • Antileukocyte recipient antibodies directed against donor WBCs	Temperature up to 104° F (40° C), chills, headache, facial flushing, palpitations, cough, chest tightness, increased pulse rate, flank pain
Hemolytic • ABO or Rh incompatibility • Intradonor incompatibility • Improper crossmatching • Improperly stored blood	Chest pain, dyspnea, facial flushing, fever, chills, shaking, hypotension, flank pain, hemoglobinuria, oliguria, bloody oozing at the infusion site or surgical incision site, burning sensation along vein receiving blood, shock, renal failure
Plasma protein incompatibility • Immunoglobulin-A incompatibility	Abdominal pain, diarrhea, dyspnea, chills, fever, flushing, hypotension

Nursing interventions
• Stop transfusion.
• Assess patient.
• Notify doctor.
• Follow facility policy.

Managing shock

Type	Pathophysiology	Causes	Physical findings	Treatment
Anaphylactic	• Edema • Blood vessel dilation • Bronchospasms • Fluid shifts	• Allergic reaction to antigens	• Pale, cool skin • Hypotension, • Respiratory distress, edema, rash	• Epinephrine • Corticosteroids • Antihistamines • I.V. fluids • Oxygen
Cardiogenic	• Decreased cardiac output (CO) • Left ventricular dysfunction • Sympathetic compensation • Myocardial ischemia	• MI • Myocardial ischemia • Myocarditis • Papillary muscle cystunction • Ventricular septal defect • Ventricular aneurysm • Acute mitral or aortic insufficiency	• Pale, cold, clammy skin • Decreased sensorium • Rapid, thready pulse • Rapid, shallow respirations • Mean arterial pressure < 60 mm Hg (adults) • Gallop rhythm, faint heart sounds	• Vasopressors • Inotropics • Vasoconstrictors • Osmotic diuretics • Oxygen • Intra-aortic balloon pump • Analgesics, sedatives
Hypovolemic	• Reduced venous return to heart due to lost fluid • Decreased ventricular filling • Decreased CO • Tissue anoxia, metabolic acidosis	• Acute blood loss • Intestinal obstruction • Burns • Peritonitis • Acute pancreatitis • Ascites • Dehydration	• Pale, cool, clammy skin • Decreased sensorium • Rapid, shallow respirations • Urine output < 20 ml/hr • Rapid, thready pulse • Mean arterial pressure < 60 mm Hg (adults) • Orthostatic vital signs	• Prompt, vigorous blood and fluid replacement • Positive inotropes • Possible diuretics

(continued)

Managing shock (continued)

Type	Pathophysiology	Causes	Physical findings	Treatment
Neurogenic	• Severe vasodilatation	• Anesthesia • Spinal cord injury	• Pale, warm, dry skin • Bounding pulse • Bradycardia • Hypotension	• I.V. fluids • Oxygen • Vasopressors • Lying flat
Septic	• Activation of chemical mediators in response to invading organisms • Functional hypovolemia	• Any pathogenic organism • Gram-negative bacteria	*Early:* • Pink, flushed skin • Rapid, shallow respirations • Rapid, full bounding pulse • Blood pressure normal to slightly elevated *Late:* • Pale, cyanotic skin • Rapid, shallow respirations • Rapid, weak, thready pulse • Hypotension	• Antimicrobial • Colloids or crystalloids • Oxygen • Diuretics • Vasopressors

Signs of increased ICP

Assessment area	Early signs	Late signs
Level of consciousness	• Increased stimulation needed • Subtle orientation loss • Restlessness and anxiety • Sudden quietness	• Unarousable
Pupils	• Pupil changes on side of lesion • One pupil constricts but then dilates (unilateral hippus) • Sluggish reaction of both pupils • Unequal pupils	• Pupils fixed and dilated or "blown"
Motor response	• Sudden weakness • Motor changes on side opposite the lesion • Positive pronator drift: With palms up, one hand pronates	• Profound weakness
Vital signs	• Intermittent increases in blood pressure	• Increased systolic pressure, widening pulse pressure, bradycardia, and abnormal respirations (Cushing's triad)

Cardiac conduction system

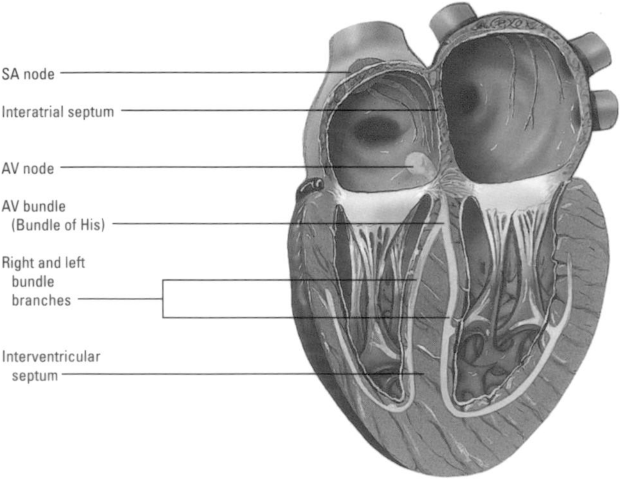

SA node

Interatrial septum

AV node

AV bundle
(Bundle of His)

Right and left
bundle
branches

Interventricular
septum

ECG grid

This ECG grid shows the horizontal axis and vertical axis and their respective measurement values.

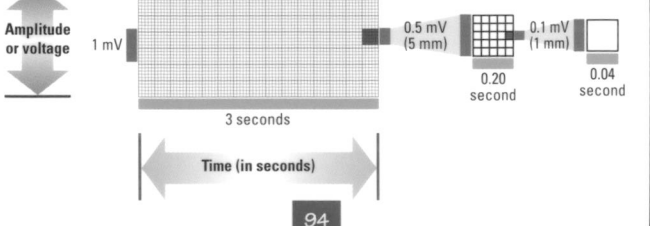

Amplitude
or voltage

1 mV

3 seconds

Time (in seconds)

0.5 mV
(5 mm)

0.20
second

0.1 mV
(1 mm)

0.04
second

Lead placement

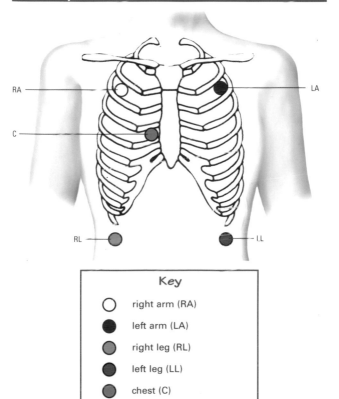

RA

LA

C

RL

LL

Key

○ right arm (RA)

● left arm (LA)

● right leg (RL)

● left leg (LL)

● chest (C)

ECG

Interpreting rhythm strips

Interpreting a rhythm strip is a skill developed through practice. You can use several methods, as long as you're consistent. Rhythm strip analysis requires a sequential and systematic approach. The eight-step method outlined below is such an approach.

Eight-step method

1. Determine the rhythm.
2. Determine the rate.
3. Evaluate the P wave.
4. Measure the PR interval.
5. Determine the QRS duration.
6. Examine the T waves.
7. Measure the QT interval.
8. Check for ectopic beats and other abnormalities.

Normal ECG

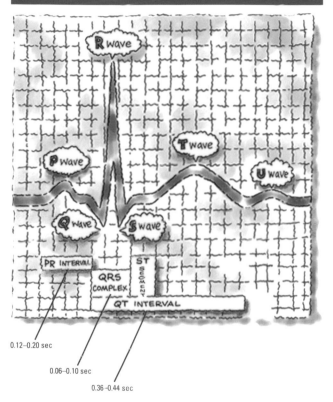

0.12–0.20 sec

0.06–0.10 sec

0.36–0.44 sec

Calculating heart rate

This table can help make the sequencing method of determining heart rate more precise. After counting the number of blocks between R waves, use this table to find the rate.

For example, if you count 20 small blocks or 4 large blocks between R waves, the rate is 75 beats/minute. To calculate the atrial rate, use the same method with P waves.

Rapid estimation

This rapid-rate calculation is also called the *countdown method*. Using the number of large blocks between R waves or P waves as a guide, you can rapidly estimate ventricular or atrial rates by memorizing the sequence "300, 150, 100, 75, 60, 50."

Number of small blocks	Heart rate
5 (1 large block)	300
6	250
7	214
8	188
9	167
10 (2 large blocks)	150
11	136
12	125
13	115
14	107
15 (3 large blocks)	100
16	94
17	88
18	83
19	79
20 (4 large blocks)	75
21	71
22	68
23	65
24	63
25 (5 large blocks)	60
26	58
27	56
28	54
29	52
30 (6 large blocks)	50
31	48
32	47
33	45
34	44
35 (7 large blocks)	43
36	42
37	41
38	39
39	38
40 (8 large blocks)	37

Normal sinus rhythm

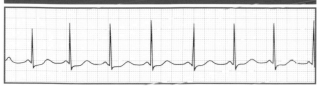

Rhythm . . . . regular
Rate . . . . 60 to 100 beats/minute
P wave . . . . normal, upright
PR interval . . . . . . 0.12 to 0.20 second
QRS complex . . . 0.06 to 0.10 second

Sinus bradycardia

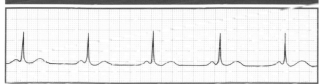

Rhythm . . . . regular
Rate . . . . <60 beats/minute
P wave . . . . normal
PR interval . . . . . . 0.12 to 0.20 second
QRS complex . . . 0.06 to 0.10 second

Sinus tachycardia

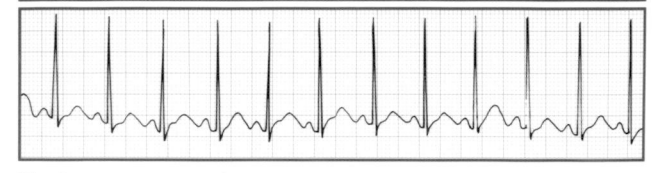

Rhythm . . . . regular
Rate . . . . 100 to 160 beats/minute
P wave . . . . normal
PR interval . . . . . . 0.12 to 0.20 second
QRS complex . . . 0.06 to 0.10 second

Premature atrial contractions (PACs)

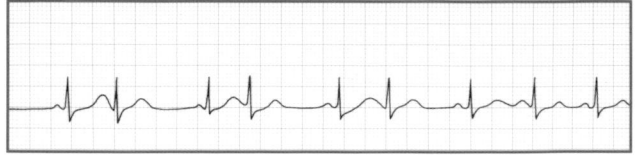

Rhythm . . . . irregular
Rate . . . . varies with underlying rhythm
P wave . . . . premature and abnormally shaped with PACs
PR interval . . . . . . usually within normal limits; varies depending on
                       ectopic focus
QRS complex . . . 0.06 to 0.10 second

Atrial tachycardia

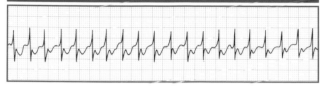

Rhythm . . . . regular
Rate . . . . atrial—150 to 250 beats/minute
                       ventricular—depends on AV conduction ratio
P wave . . . . hidden in the preceding T wave
PR interval . . . . . . not visible
QRS complex . . . 0.06 to 0 10 second

Atrial flutter

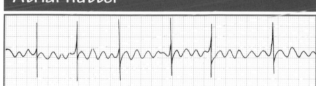

Rhythm . . . . atrial—regular
                       ventricular—typically irregular
Rate . . . . atrial—250 to 400 beats/minute
                       ventricular—usually 60 to 100 beats/minute;
                       depends on degree of AV block
P wave . . . . classic sawtooth appearance
PR interval . . . . . . unmeasurable
QRS complex . . . 0.06 to 0.10 second

Atrial fibrillation

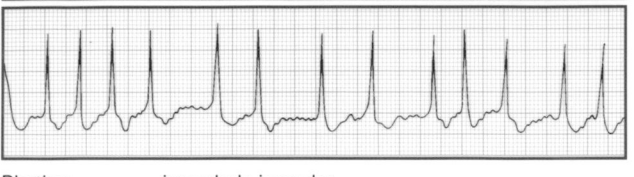

Rhythm . . . . irregularly irregular
Rate . . . . atrial—usually > 400 beats/minute
ventricular—varies
P wave . . . . absent; replaced by fine fibrillatory waves,
or f waves
PR interval . . . . . . indiscernible
QRS complex . . . 0.06 to 0.10 second

Premature junctional contractions (PJCs)

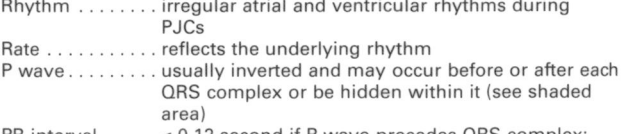

Rhythm . . . . irregular atrial and ventricular rhythms during
PJCs
Rate . . . . reflects the underlying rhythm
P wave . . . . usually inverted and may occur before or after each
QRS complex or be hidden within it (see shaded
area)
PR interval . . . . . . < 0.12 second if P wave precedes QRS complex;
otherwise unmeasurable
QRS complex . . . 0.06 to 0.10 second

Junctional escape rhythm

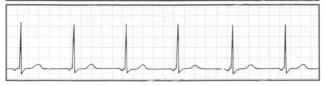

Rhythm . . . . regular
Rate . . . . 40 to 60 beats/minute
P wave . . . . usually inverted and may occur before or after each
                   QRS complex or be hidden within it
PR interval . . . . . . < 0.12 second if P wave precedes QRS complex;
                   otherwise unmeasurable
QRS complex . . . 0.10 second

Accelerated junctional rhythm

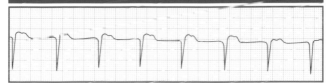

Rhythm . . . . regular
Rate . . . . 60 to 100 beats/minute
P wave . . . . usually inverted and may occur before or after each
                   QRS complex or be hidden within it
PR interval . . . . . . < 0.12 second if P wave precedes QRS complex;
                   otherwise unmeasurable
QRS complex . . . 0.06 to 0.10 second

Premature ventricular contractions (PVCs)

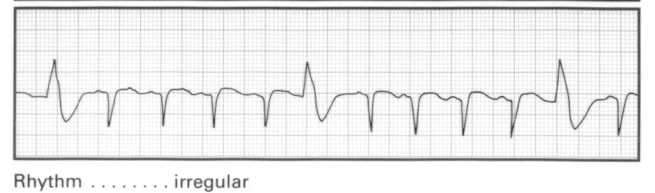

Rhythm . . . . irregular
Rate . . . . reflects the underlying rhythm
P wave . . . . none with PVC, but P wave present with other QRS
                  complexes
PR interval . . . . . . unmeasurable except in underlying rhythm
QRS complex . . . early, with bizarre configuration and duration of
                  > 0.12 second; QRS complexes are normal in under-
                  lying rhythm

Ventricular tachycardia

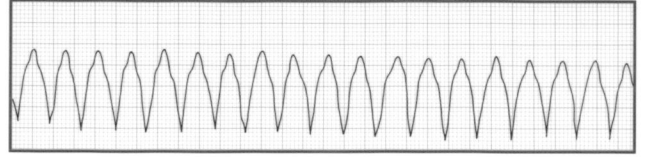

Rhythm . . . . regular
Rate . . . . atrial—can't be determined
                  ventricular—100 to 250 beats/minute
P wave . . . . absent
PR interval . . . . . . unmeasurable
QRS complex . . . > 0.12 second; wide and bizarre

Ventricular fibrillation

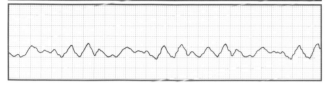

Rhythm . . . . chaotic
Rate , ... can't be determined
P wave . . . . absent
PR interval . . . . . . unmeasurable
QRS complex . . . indiscernible

Asystole

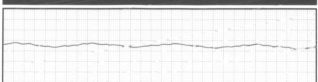

Rhythm . . . . atrial—usually indiscernible
ventricular— no rhythm
Rate . . . . atrial—usually indiscernible
ventricular—no rate
P wave . . . . may be present
PR interval . . . . . . unmeasurable
QRS complex . . . absent or occasional escape beats

First-degree atrioventricular block

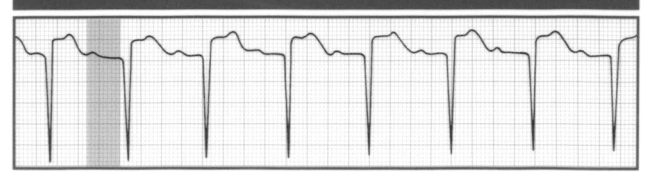

Rhythm . . . . regular
Rate . . . . within normal limits
P wave. . . . . normal
PR interval. . . . . . > 0.20 second (see shaded area) but constant
QRS complex . . . 0.06 to 0.10 second

Type I second-degree atrioventricular block

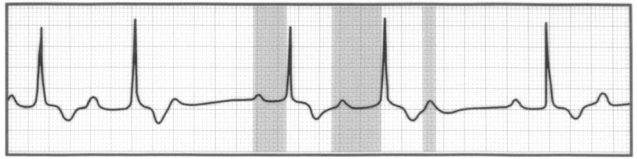

Rhythm . . . . atrial—regular
                       ventricular—irregular
Rate . . . . atrial—exceeds ventricular rate;
                       both remain within normal limits
P wave. . . . . normal
PR interval. . . . . . progressively prolonged (see shaded areas) until a
                       P wave appears without a QRS complex
QRS complex . . . 0.06 to 0.10 second

Type II second-degree atrioventricular block

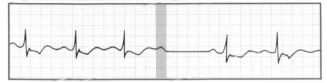

Rhythm .... atrial—regular
            ventricular—irregular
Rate .... atrial—within normal limits
            ventricular—slower than atrial but may be within
            normal limits
P wave......... normal
PR interval..... constant for conducted beats
QRS complex ... within normal limits; absent for dropped beats

Third-degree atrioventricular block

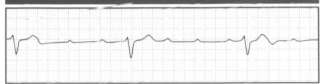

Rhythm .... regular
Rate .... atria and ventricles beat independently
            atrial—60 to 100 beats/minute
            ventricular—40 to 60 beats/minute if intranodal
            block; < 40 beats/minute if infranodal block
P wave......... normal
PR interval...... varied; not applicable or measurable
QRS complex ... normal or widened

Cancer detection screening

This health maintenance schedule is recommended for adult patients older than age 18.

Evaluation	Recommendations
Breast	
• Clinical breast examination	• Every year for women age 40 and older
	• Every 3 years for women ages 20 to 39
• Mammogram	• Every year for women age 40 and older
• Breast self-examination	• Monthly for women age 20 and older (optional)
Cervix	
• Papanicolaou (Pap) test	• All women should begin cervical cancer screening 3 years after they begin to have vaginal intercourse, but no later than age 21
	• Annually for women beginning at age 21
	• Beginning at age 30, every 2 to 3 years after three or more consecutive satisfactory examinations with normal findings
	• May stop in women age 70 and older with three or more consecutive examinations and no abnormal Pap test in the past 10 years
Endometrium	
For all women at risk for hereditary nonpolyposis colon cancer	
• Tissue sampling	• Annually, beginning at age 35

(continued)

Cancer detection screening *(continued)*

Evaluation	Recommendations

Colon and rectum (one of the examinations below)
For men and women age 50 and older

• Fecal occult blood test (FOBT)	• Every year
• Flexible sigmoidoscopy	• Every 5 years
• FOBT plus flexible sigmoidoscopy	• FOBT every year plus flexible sigmoidoscopy every 5 years (preferred by clinicians over either of two alone)
• Colonoscopy	• Every 10 years
• Double-contrast barium enema	• Every 5 years

Prostate
For men age 50 and older with life expectancy of at least 10 years and younger men at high risk at age 45

• Prostate-specific antigen	• Annually
• Digital rectal examination	• Annually

Testicular

• Testicular examination	• Annually
• Testicular self-examination	• Monthly, particularly for men between ages 15 and 40, who are at higher risk

The ABCDEs of malignant melanoma

A simple **ABCDE** rule outlines the warning signs of malignant melanoma:

A is for asymmetry: One half of a mole or birthmark doesn't match the other.

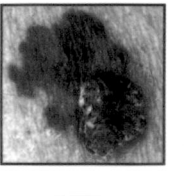

B is for border: The edges are irregular, ragged, notched, or blurred.

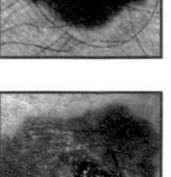

C is for color: The pigmentation isn't uniform but may have varying degrees of brown or black, or sometimes red.

D is for diameter greater than 1″ (0.6 cm): Any sudden or progressive increase in size should be of concern.

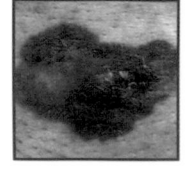

E is for elevation: If a mole is elevated, or raised from the skin, it should be considered suspicious.

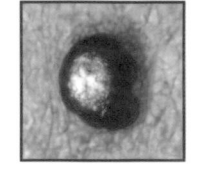

Heart valves

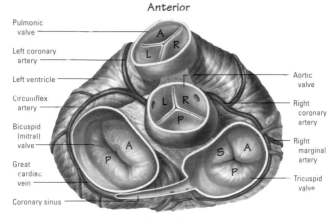

Anterior

Pulmonic valve

Left coronary artery

Left ventricle

Circumflex artery

Bicuspid (mitral) valve

Great cardiac vein

Coronary sinus

Aortic valve

Right coronary artery

Right marginal artery

Tricuspid valve

Posterior

Key

A Anterior
P Posterior
L Left
R Right
S Septal

Teaching

Heart and coronary vessels

Anterior view

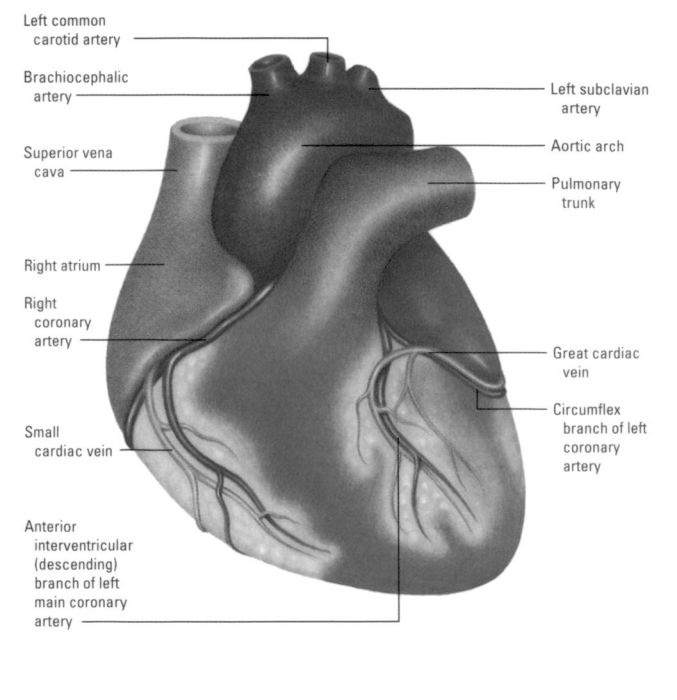

Left common
carotid artery

Brachiocephalic
artery

Superior vena
cava

Right atrium

Right
coronary
artery

Small
cardiac vein

Anterior
interventricular
(descending)
branch of left
main coronary
artery

Left subclavian
artery

Aortic arch

Pulmonary
trunk

Great cardiac
vein

Circumflex
branch of left
coronary
artery

Heart and coronary vessels (continued)

Posterior view

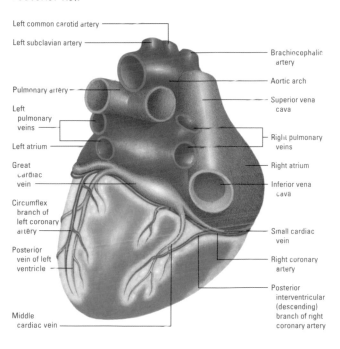

Left common carotid artery

Left subclavian artery

Pulmonary artery

Left pulmonary veins

Left atrium

Great cardiac vein

Circumflex branch of left coronary artery

Posterior vein of left ventricle

Middle cardiac vein

Brachiocephalic artery

Aortic arch

Superior vena cava

Right pulmonary veins

Right atrium

Inferior vena cava

Small cardiac vein

Right coronary artery

Posterior interventricular (descending) branch of right coronary artery

Teaching

Thrombus formation

The most common cause of acute coronary syndrome is thrombus formation and subsequent coronary artery occlusion.

The first step in thrombus formation involves plaque rupture (below top left). As platelets adhere to the damaged area, they're exposed to activating factors, including collagen, thrombin, and von Willebrand (VW) factor (below top right).

Activation of the exposed platelets causes expression of glycoprotein IIb/IIIa receptors that bind fibrinogen (below bottom left). This, in turn, leads to further platelet aggregation and adhesion, enlarging the thrombus (below bottom right).

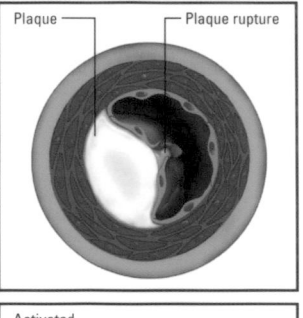

Plaque — Plaque rupture

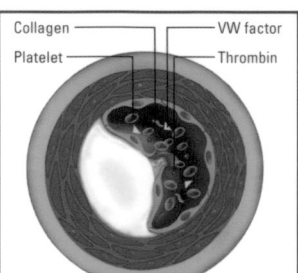

Collagen — VW factor
Platelet — Thrombin

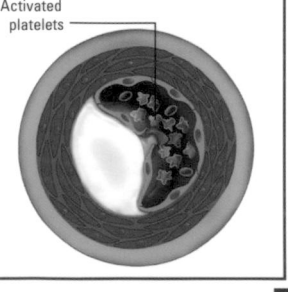

Activated platelets

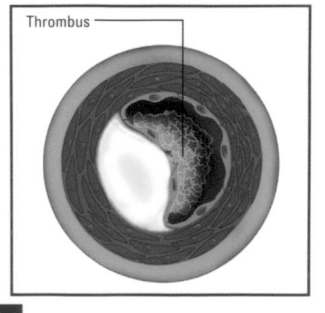

Thrombus

Looking at angioplasty

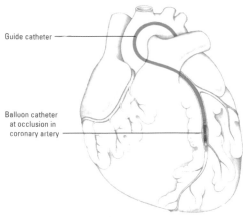

Guide catheter

Balloon catheter at occlusion in coronary artery

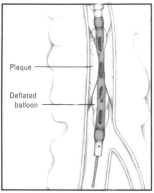

Plaque

Deflated balloon

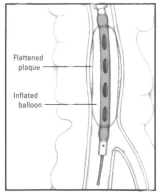

Flattened plaque

Inflated balloon

Teaching

Respiratory tract

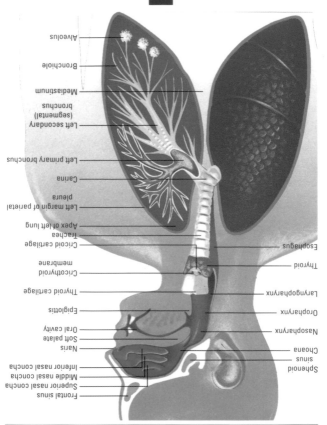

- Frontal sinus
- Superior nasal concha
- Middle nasal concha
- Inferior nasal concha
- Naris
- Soft palate
- Oral cavity
- Epiglottis
- Thyroid cartilage
- Cricothyroid membrane
- Cricoid cartilage
- Trachea
- Apex of left lung
- Left margin of parietal pleura
- Carina
- Left primary bronchus
- Left secondary (segmental) bronchus
- Mediastinum
- Bronchiole
- Alveolus

- Sphenoid sinus
- Choana
- Nasopharynx
- Oropharynx
- Laryngopharynx
- Thyroid
- Esophagus

GI system

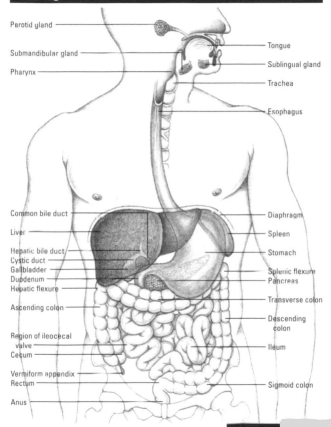

- Parotid gland
- Submandibular gland
- Pharynx
- Tongue
- Sublingual gland
- Trachea
- Esophagus
- Common bile duct
- Liver
- Hepatic bile duct
- Cystic duct
- Gallbladder
- Duodenum
- Hepatic flexure
- Ascending colon
- Region of ileocecal valve
- Cecum
- Vermiform appendix
- Rectum
- Anus
- Diaphragm
- Spleen
- Stomach
- Splenic flexure
- Pancreas
- Transverse colon
- Descending colon
- Ileum
- Sigmoid colon

Teaching

Urinary tract

Anterior view

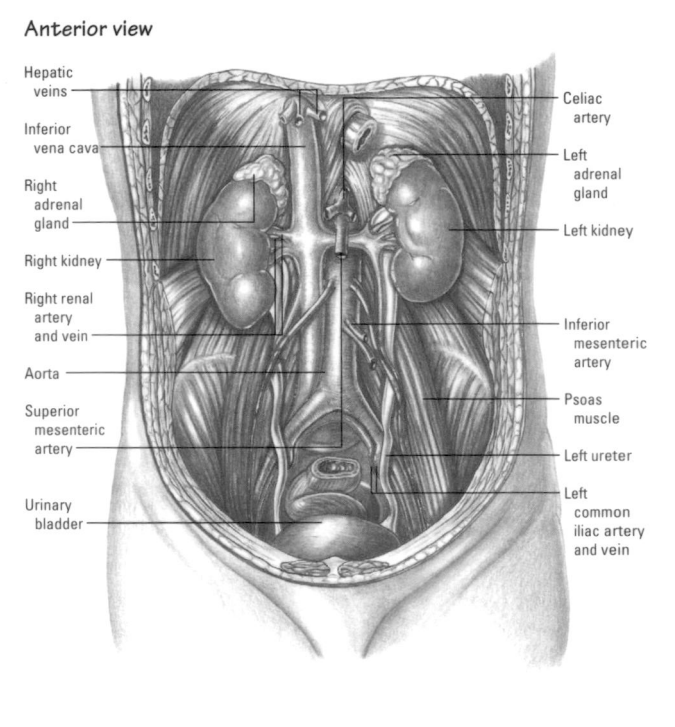

Hepatic veins

Inferior vena cava

Right adrenal gland

Right kidney

Right renal artery and vein

Aorta

Superior mesenteric artery

Urinary bladder

Celiac artery

Left adrenal gland

Left kidney

Inferior mesenteric artery

Psoas muscle

Left ureter

Left common iliac artery and vein

CONVERSION FACTORS

Weight conversion

To convert a patient's weight in pounds to kilograms, divide the number of pounds by 2.2 kg; to convert a patient's weight in kilograms to pounds, multiply the number of kilograms by 2.2 lb.

Pounds	Kilograms
10	4.5
20	9
30	13.6
40	18.1
50	22.7
60	27.2
70	31.8
80	36.3
90	40.9
100	45.4
110	49.9
120	54.4
130	59
140	63.5
150	68
160	72.6
170	77.1
180	81.6
190	86.2
200	90.8
210	95.5
220	100
230	104.5
240	109.1
250	113.6
260	118.2
270	122.7
280	127.3
290	131.8
300	136.4

Temperature conversion

To convert Fahrenheit to Celsius, subtract 32 from the temperature in Fahrenheit and then divide by 1.8; to convert Celsius to Fahrenheit, multiply the temperature in Celsius by 1.8 and then add 32.

$$(F - 32) \div 1.8 = \text{degrees Celsius}$$

$$(C \times 1.8) + 32 = \text{degrees Fahrenheit}$$

Degrees Fahrenheit (°F)	Degrees Celsius (°C)	Degrees Fahrenheit (°F)	Degrees Celsius (°C)
89.6	32	100.8	38.2
91.4	33	101	38.3
93.2	34	101.2	38.4
94.3	34.6	101.4	38.6
95.0	35	101.8	38.8
95.4	35.2	102	38.9
96.2	35.7	102.2	39
96.8	36	102.6	39.2
97.2	36.2	102.8	39.3
97.6	36.4	103	39.4
98	36.7	103.2	39.6
98.6	37	103.4	39.7
99	37.2	103.6	39.8
99.3	37.4	104	40
99.7	37.6	104.4	40.2
100	37.8	104.6	40.3
100.4	38	104.8	40.4
		105	40.6

Solid equivalents

Milligram (mg)	Gram (g)	Grain (Gr)
1,000	1	15
600 (or 650)	0.6	10
500	0.5	7.5
300 (or 325)	0.3	5
200	0.2	3
100	0.1	1.5
60 (or 65)	0.06	1
30	0.03	½
15	0.15	¼

Liquid equivalents

Metric (ml)	Apothecary	Household
	1 minim = 1 gtt	—
1	16 minims	—
4	1 dram	—
5	—	1 tsp
15	4 drams or ½ ounce	1 tbs
30	8 drams or 1 ounce	1 ounce or 2 tbs
50	—	1 pint
1,000	—	1 quart or 2 pints

INFECTION CONTROL

Standard precautions

These guidelines were developed by the Centers for Disease Control and Prevention (CDC) to provide the widest possible protection against the transmission of infection. CDC officials recommend that health care workers handle all blood, body fluids, tissues, and contact with mucous membranes and broken skin as if they contained infectious agents, regardless of the patient's diagnosis.

Implementation

• Wash your hands before and after patient care, after removing gloves, or immediately after contamination with blood, body fluid, excretions, secretions, or drainage.
• Wear gloves if you will or could come in contact with blood, specimens, tissue, body fluids, secretions, excretions, mucous membranes, broken skin, or contaminated objects or surfaces.
• Change gloves and wash your hands between patients or if you touch anything with a high concentration of microorganisms when caring for the same patient.
• Wear a fluid-resistant gown, eye protection, and mask during procedures that are likely to generate droplets of blood or body fluids.

• Carefully handle used patient care equipment that is soiled with blood or body fluids. Follow facility guidelines for cleaning and disinfection of equipment and environmental surfaces.
• Keep contaminated linens away from your body and place in properly labeled containers.
• Handle needles and sharps carefully and immediately discard in an impervious disposal box after use. Use sharps with safety features whenever possible.
• Immediately notify your supervisor of a needle-stick or sharp instrument injury, mucosal splash, or contamination of nonintact skin with blood or body fluids to initiate appropriate investigation of the incident and care.
• Use mouthpieces, resuscitation bags, or ventilation devices in place of mouth-to mouth resuscitation.
• Place the patient who can't maintain hygiene measures or who may contaminate the environment in a private room.
• If occupational exposure to blood is likely, get the HBV vaccine series.
• Become familiar with your facility's infection control policies and procedures.

Transmission-based precautions

Whenever a patient is known or suspected to be infected with a highly contagious or epidemiologically important pathogen that's transmitted by air, droplet, or contact with dry skin or other contaminated surfaces, follow transmission-based precautions *in addition to* standard precautions.

Airborne precautions

Follow these precautions, in addition to standard precautions:
• Place the patient in a private room that has monitored negative air pressure in relation to surrounding areas and keep the door closed.
• Respiratory protection must be worn by all persons entering the room. Such protection is provided by a disposable respirator (N-95 respirator or high-efficiency particulate air respirator) or a reusable respirator (powered air-purifying respirator).
• Limit patient transport and movement out of the room. If the patient must leave the room, he must wear a surgical mask.

Droplet precautions

Follow these precautions, in addition to standard precautions:
• Place the patient in a private room.
• Wear a mask when working within 3 ft of the infected patient. For a patient with known tuberculosis, wear a disposable or reusable respirator.
• Instruct visitors to wear a mask if within 3 ft of the patient.
• Limit patient transport and movement out of the room. If the patient must leave the room, he must wear a surgical mask.

Contact precautions

Follow these precautions, in addition to standard precautions:
• Place the patient in a private room.
• Wear gloves whenever you enter the patient's room. Always change gloves after contact with infected material. Remove gloves before leaving the room. Wash your hands with an antimicrobial soap or use a waterless antiseptic immediately after removing gloves and avoid touching contaminated surfaces.
• Wear a fluid-resistant gown when entering the patient's room if you think your clothing will become contaminated by contact, blood, or body fluids. Remove the gown before leaving the room.
• Limit patient transport and movement out of the room. If the patient must leave the room, he must wear a surgical mask.

NANDA nursing diagnoses

Here's a list of the 2005-2006 nursing diagnosis classifications according to their domains. New nursing diagnoses include: Impaired religiosity, Readiness for enhanced religiosity, Risk for dysfunctional grieving, Risk for impaired religiosity, and Sedentary lifestyle.

Domain: Health promotion

- Effective therapeutic regimen management
- Health-seeking behaviors (specify)
- Impaired home maintenance
- Ineffective community therapeutic regimen management
- Ineffective family therapeutic regimen management
- Ineffective health maintenance
- Ineffective therapeutic regimen management
- Readiness for enhanced management of therapeutic regimen
- Readiness for enhanced nutrition

Domain: Nutrition

- Deficient fluid volume
- Excess fluid volume
- Imbalanced nutrition: Less than body requirements
- Imbalanced nutrition: More than body requirements
- Impaired swallowing
- Ineffective infant feeding pattern
- Readiness for enhanced fluid balance
- Risk for deficient fluid volume
- Risk for imbalanced fluid volume
- Risk for imbalanced nutrition: More than body requirements

Domain: Elimination and exchange

- Bowel incontinence
- Constipation
- Diarrhea
- Functional urinary incontinence
- Impaired gas exchange
- Impaired urinary elimination
- Perceived constipation
- Readiness for enhanced urinary elimination
- Reflex urinary incontinence
- Risk for constipation
- Risk for urge urinary incontinence
- Stress urinary incontinence
- Total urinary incontinence
- Urge urinary incontinence
- Urinary retention

Domain: Activity/Rest

- Activity intolerance
- Bathing or hygiene self-care deficit
- Decreased cardiac output
- Deficient diversional activity
- Delayed surgical recovery
- Disturbed sleep pattern

NANDA nursing diagnoses (continued)

Domain: Activity/Rest

(continued)

- Dressing or grooming self-care deficit
- Dysfunctional ventilatory weaning response
- Energy field disturbance
- Fatigue
- Feeding self-care deficit
- Impaired bed mobility
- Impaired physical mobility
- Impaired spontaneous ventilation
- Impaired transfer ability
- Impaired walking
- Impaired wheelchair mobility
- Ineffective breathing pattern
- Ineffective tissue perfusion (specify type: renal, cerebral, cardiopulmonary, gastrointestinal, peripheral)
- Readiness for enhanced sleep
- Risk for activity intolerance
- Risk for disuse syndrome
- Sedentary lifestyle
- Sleep deprivation
- Toileting self-care deficit

Domain: Perception/Cognition

- Acute confusion
- Chronic confusion
- Deficient knowledge (specify)
- Disturbed sensory perception (specify: visual, auditory, kinesthetic, gustatory, tactile, olfactory)
- Disturbed thought processes
- Impaired environmental interpretation syndrome
- Impaired memory
- Impaired verbal communication
- Readiness for enhanced communication
- Readiness for enhanced knowledge (specify)
- Unilateral neglect
- Wandering

Domain: Self-perception

- Chronic low self-esteem
- Disturbed body image
- Disturbed personal identity
- Hopelessness
- Powerlessness
- Readiness for enhanced self-concept
- Risk for loneliness
- Risk for powerlessness
- Risk for situational low self-esteem
- Situational low self-esteem

Domain: Role relationships

- Caregiver role strain
- Dysfunctional family processes: Alcoholism
- Effective breast-feeding
- Impaired parenting
- Impaired social interaction
- Ineffective breast-feeding
- Ineffective role performance
- Interrupted breast-feeding
- Interrupted family processes

(continued)

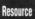

Resource

NANDA nursing diagnoses *(continued)*

Domain: Role relationships

(continued)

- Parental role conflict
- Readiness for enhanced family processes
- Readiness for enhanced parenting
- Risk for caregiver role strain
- Risk for impaired parent/infant/child attachment
- Risk for impaired parenting

Domain: Sexuality

- Ineffective sexuality pattern
- Sexual dysfunction

Domain: Coping/Stress tolerance

- Anticipatory grieving
- Anxiety
- Autonomic dysreflexia
- Chronic sorrow
- Compromised family coping
- Death anxiety
- Decreased intracranial adaptive capacity
- Defensive coping
- Disabled family coping
- Disorganized infant behavior
- Dysfunctional grieving
- Fear
- Impaired adjustment
- Ineffective community coping
- Ineffective coping
- Ineffective denial
- Posttrauma syndrome
- Rape-trauma syndrome

- Rape-trauma syndrome: Compound reaction
- Rape-trauma syndrome: Silent reaction
- Readiness for enhanced community coping
- Readiness for enhanced family coping
- Readiness for enhanced individual coping
- Readiness for enhanced organized infant behavior
- Relocation stress syndrome
- Risk for autonomic dysreflexia
- Risk for disorganized infant behavior
- Risk for dysfunctional grieving
- Risk for posttrauma syndrome
- Risk for relocation stress syndrome

Domain: Life principles

- Decisional conflict (specify)
- Impaired religiosity
- Noncompliance (specify)
- Readiness for enhanced religiosity
- Readiness for enhanced spiritual well-being
- Risk for impaired religiosity
- Risk for spiritual distress
- Spiritual distress

Domain: Safety/Protection

- Hyperthermia
- Hypothermia
- Impaired dentition

NANDA nursing diagnoses (continued)

Domain: Safety/Protection

(continued)

- Impaired oral mucous membrane
- Impaired skin integrity
- Impaired tissue integrity
- Ineffective airway clearance
- Ineffective protection
- Ineffective thermoregulation
- Latex allergy response
- Risk for aspiration
- Risk for falls
- Risk for imbalanced body temperature
- Risk for impaired skin integrity
- Risk for infection
- Risk for injury
- Risk for latex allergy response
- Risk for other-directed violence
- Risk for perioperative-positioning injury
- Risk for peripheral neurovascular dysfunction
- Risk for poisoning
- Risk for self-directed violence
- Risk for self-mutilation
- Risk for sudden infant death syndrome
- Risk for suffocation
- Risk for suicide
- Risk for trauma
- Self-mutilation

Domain: Comfort

- Acute pain
- Chronic pain
- Nausea
- Social isolation

Domain: Growth/Development

- Adult failure to thrive
- Delayed growth and development
- Risk for delayed development
- Risk for disproportionate growth

© NANDA International (2005). *NANDA Nursing Diagnoses: Definitions and Classifications 2005-2006.* Philadelphia: NANDA. Reprinted with permission.

Cultural considerations in patient care

As a health care professional you'll interact with a diverse, multicultural patient population. Each culture has its own unique set of beliefs about health and illness and dietary practices that you need to know when providing care.

Cultural group	Health and illness philosophy	Dietary practices
African Americans	• May believe illness is related to supernatural causes, such as punishment from God or an evil spell • Believe health is a feeling of well-being • May seek advice and remedies from faith or folk healers	• May have food restrictions based on religious beliefs, such as not eating pork if Muslim • May view cooked greens as good for health
Arab Americans	• Believe health is a gift from God and that one should care for self by eating right and minimizing stressors • May believe illness is caused by the evil eye, bad luck, stress, or an imbalance between hot and cold or moist and dry • May assume passive role as patient • May use amulets to ward off evil eye during illness • Believe in complete rest and relieving self of all responsibilities during an illness • Tend to express pain vocally; may have low pain threshold	• Don't mix milk and fish, sweet and sour, or hot and cold • Don't use ice in drinks; believe hot soup can help recovery • If Muslim, prohibited from drinking alcohol and eating pork or ham

(continued)

Cultural considerations in patient care
(continued)

Cultural group	Health and illness philosophy	Dietary practices
Chinese Americans	• Believe health is a balance of Yin and Yang; illness stems from an imbalance of these elements; health requires harmony between body, mind, and spirit • May use herbalists or acupuncturists before seeking medical help • May use good luck objects, such as jade or rope tied around waist • Family expected to take care of patient, who assumes a passive role • Tend not to readily express pain; stoic by nature	• Staples are rice, noodles, and vegetables; tend to use chopsticks • Choose foods to help balance the Yin (cold) and Yang (hot) • Drink hot liquids, especially when sick
Japanese Americans	• Believe that health is a balance of oneself, society, and the universe • May believe illness is karma, resulting from behavior in present or past life • May believe certain food combinations cause illness • May not complain of symptoms until severe	• Eat rice with most meals; may use chopsticks • Diet high in salt and low in sugar, fat, animal protein, and cholesterol
Mexican Americans	• Believe that health is influenced by environment, fate, and God's will • May believe in Galen's theory that the four humors in the body — blood, phlegm, yellow bile, and black bile — must be kept in balance • May use herbal teas and soup to aid in recuperation • May express pain by nonverbal cues • Family may want to keep seriousness of illness from patient	• Beans and tortillas are staples • Eat lots of fresh fruits and vegetables

Cultural considerations in patient care
(continued)

Cultural group	Health and illness philosophy	Dietary practices
Native Americans	• Use herbs and roots; each tribe has its own unique medicinal practices • Most use modern medicine where available • The Medicine Wheel is an ancient symbol used • For some, 4 is a sacred number, associated with the four primary laws of creation: Life, Unity, Equality, and Eternity • May use tobacco for important religious, ceremonial, and medicinal purposes; may sprinkle it around the bed of sick people to protect and heal them	• Have balanced diet of seafood, fruits, greens, corn, rice, and garden vegetables; salt consumption is low • Specific dietary practices are based on location; urban dwellers often eat most types of meat, while rural dwellers often consume only lamb and goat

NUTRITION

Troubleshooting tube feeding problems

Complication	Nursing interventions
Aspiration of gastric secretions	• Discontinue feeding immediately. • Perform tracheal suction of aspirated contents. • Notify the doctor. • Check tube placement before feeding to prevent complication.
Tube obstruction	• Flush the tube with warm water. If necessary, replace the tube. • Flush the tube with 50 ml of water after each feeding to remove excess sticky formula, which could occlude the tube.
Oral, nasal, or pharyngeal irritation or necrosis	• Provide frequent oral hygiene. • Change the tube's position. If necessary, replace the tube.
Vomiting, bloating, diarrhea, or cramps	• Reduce the flow rate. • Administer metoclopramide to increase GI motility. • Warm the formula to prevent GI distress. • For 30 minutes after feeding, position the patient on his right side with his head elevated to facilitate gastric emptying. • Notify the doctor.
Constipation	• Provide additional fluids if the patient can tolerate them. • Administer a bulk-forming laxative. • Increase the fruit, vegetable, or sugar content of the feeding.
Electrolyte imbalance	• Monitor serum electrolyte levels. • Notify the doctor. He may want to adjust the formula content to correct the deficiency.
Hyperglycemia	• Monitor blood glucose levels; notify the doctor of elevated levels. • Administer insulin if ordered. • The doctor may adjust the glucose content of the formula.

Resource

Evaluating nutritional disorders

Body system or region	Sign or symptom	Implications
General	• Weakness and fatigue	• Anemia, electrolyte imbalance
	• Weight loss	• Decreased calorie intake, increased calorie use, or inadequate nutrient intake or absorption
Skin, hair, and nails	• Dry, flaky skin	• Vitamin A, vitamin B complex, or linoleic acid deficiency
	• Rough, scaly skin with bumps	• Vitamin A deficiency
	• Petechiae or ecchymoses	• Vitamin C or K deficiency
	• Sore that won't heal	• Protein, vitamin C, or zinc deficiency
	• Thinning, dry hair	• Protein deficiency
	• Spoon-shaped, brittle, or ridged nails	• Iron deficiency
Eyes	• Night blindness; corneal swelling, softening, or dryness; Bitot's spots	• Vitamin A deficiency
	• Red conjunctiva	• Riboflavin deficiency
Throat and mouth	• Cracks at corner of mouth	• Riboflavin or niacin deficiency
	• Magenta tongue	• Riboflavin deficiency
	• Beefy, red tongue	• Vitamin B_{12} deficiency
	• Soft, spongy, bleeding gums	• Vitamin C deficiency
	• Swollen neck (goiter)	• Iodine deficiency

Evaluating nutritional disorders (continued)

Body system or region	Sign or symptom	Implications
Cardiovascular	• Edema	• Protein deficiency
	• Tachycardia, hypotension	• Fluid volume deficit
GI	• Ascites	• Protein deficiency
Musculoskeletal	• Bone pain and bow leg	• Vitamin D or calcium deficiency
	• Muscle wasting	• Protein, carbohydrate, and fat deficiency
Neurologic	• Altered mental status	• Dehydration and thiamine or vitamin B_{12} deficiency
	• Paresthesia	• Vitamin B_{12}, pyridoxine, or thiamine deficiency

Potassium-rich foods

Fruits

- Avocados
- Bananas
- Cantaloupes
- Grapefruit juice
- Honeydew melons
- Oranges
- Orange juice
- Fresh peaches
- Dried fruit

Vegetables

- Broccoli
- Greens
- Spinach
- Tomatoes
- Tomato soup
- Tomato juice

Beans

- Baked beans
- Black beans
- Black-eyed peas
- Butter beans
- Chickpeas
- Crowder peas
- Great Northern beans
- Kidney beans
- Lentils
- Lima beans
- Navy beans
- Pinto beans
- Split peas

Potatoes

- Baked white potatoes
- Baked sweet potatoes
- Potato chips
- French fries
- Instant potato mixes
- Home fries
- Yams

Miscellaneous foods

- Molasses
- Nuts
- Salt substitutes

Calcium-rich foods

Dairy

- Milk
- Yogurt
- Ice cream
- Cheese

Vegetables

- Broccoli
- Collard, turnip greens, or kale

Fruits

- Dried figs
- Orange juice with calcium added

Fish/seafood

- Oysters
- Salmon with bones
- Sardines
- Canned shrimp

Miscellaneous foods

- Dried or refried beans
- Molasses
- Tofu
- Pesto or cheese sauce

Tips to reduce sodium intake

Read labels

• Read food labels for sodium content.
• Use food products with reduced sodium or no added salt.
• Be aware that soy sauce, broth, and foods that are pickled or cured have high sodium contents.

Cook wisely

• Instead of cooking with salt, use herbs, spices, cooking wines, lemon, lime, or vinegar to enhance food flavors.
• Cook pasta and rice without salt.
• Rinse canned foods, such as tuna, to remove some sodium.
• Avoid adding salt to foods, especially at the table.
• Avoid condiments, such as soy and teriyaki sauces and mono-sodium glutamate (MSG)—or use lower-sodium versions.

Watch your diet

• Eat fresh poultry, fish, and lean meat rather than canned, smoked, or processed versions (which typically contain a lot of sodium).
• Whenever possible, eat fresh foods rather than canned or convenience foods
• Limit intake of cured foods (such as bacon and ham), foods packed in brine (pickles, olives, and sauerkraut), and condiments (mustard, ketchup, horseradish, and Worcestershire sauce).
• When dining out, ask how food is prepared. Ask that your food be prepared without added salt or MSG.

Wound dressings

Some dressings absorb moisture from a wound bed, whereas others add moisture to it. Use this chart to quickly determine the category of dressing that's appropriate for your patient.

Moisture scale

Absorb moisture		Neutral (maintain existing moisture level)		Add moisture	
• Alginates • Specialty absorptives • Vacuum-assisted closure (VAC) device • Gauze	• Foams • Hydrocolloids • Compression dressings	• Composites • Mini-VAC device	• Transparent films • Biological dressings • Collagen dressings • Contact layers • Warm-Up Therapy System	• Sheet hydrogels	• Amorphous hydrogel • Debriding agents

Choosing a wound dressing

The patient's needs and wound characteristics determine which type of dressing to use on a wound.

Gauze dressings

Gauze dressings are permeable to water, water vapor, and oxygen. When uncertain about which dressing to use, you may apply a gauze dressing moistened in saline solution until a wound specialist recommends treatment.

Hydrocolloid dressings

Hydrocolloid dressings are adhesive, moldable wafers that usually have waterproof backings. They're impermeable to oxygen, water, and water vapor. Most have some absorptive properties.

Transparent film dressings

Transparent film dressings are clear, adherent, and nonabsorptive. They are permeable to oxygen and water vapor but not to water. Their transparency allows visual inspection. They can't absorb drainage so they're used on partial thickness wounds with minimal exudate.

Alginate dressings

Alginate dressings absorb excessive exudate and may be used on infected wounds. As they absorb exudate, they turn into a gel that keeps the wound bed moist and promotes healing. When exudate is no longer excessive, switch to another type of dressing.

Foam dressings

Foam dressings are somewhat absorptive and may be adherent. They promote moist wound healing and are useful when a nonadherent surface is desired.

Hydrogel dressings

Water-based and nonadherent, hydrogel dressings have some absorptive properties. They may have a cooling effect, which eases pain, and are used when the wound needs moisture.

English-Spanish picture dictionary

crutches
muletas

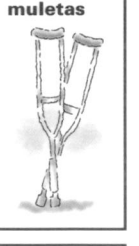

cane
bastón

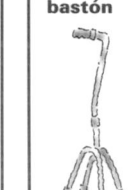

walker
andador

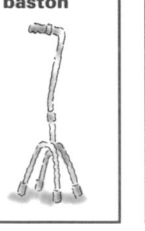

wheelchair
silla de ruedas

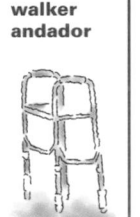

I want to sit in the chair.
Quiero sentarme en la silla.

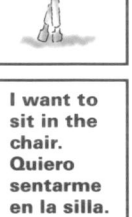

I want to go for a walk.
Quiero caminar.

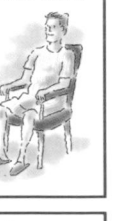

I want to see the doctor.
Quiero ver a mi médico.

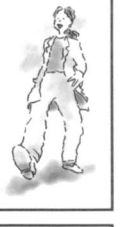

TV on
TV prendida

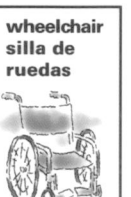

TV off
TV apagada

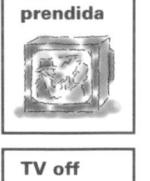

juice
jugo

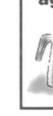

water
agua

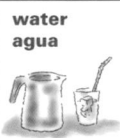

pencil and paper
lápiz y papel

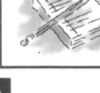

slippers
pantuflas

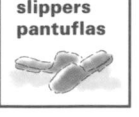

I want to get back in bed.
Quiero volver a la cama.

bed higher
cama más alta

bed lower
cama más baja

pain   dolor

mild
leve

bothersome
molesto

throbbing
pulsante

intense
intenso

I need my inhaler.
Necesito mi inhalador.

ice pack
bolsa de hielo

ice chips
edacitos de hielo

urinal
orinal

bedpan
chata

pillow
almohada

commode
cómoda

blanket
manta

hot
caliente

telephone
teléfono

cold
frío(a)

English-Spanish quick reference guide

anemia	la anemia
angina	la angina
appendicitis	la apendicitis
arteriosclerosis	la arteriosclerosis
arthritis	la artritis
asthma	el asma
backache	el dolor de espalda
blindness	la ceguera
bronchitis	la bronquitis
burn	la quemadura
(first, second, or third degree)	(de primer, segundo o tercer grado)
bursitis	la bursitis
cancer	el cáncer
chickenpox	la varicela, las viruelas locas
chills	los escalofríos
cold	el catarro, el resfriado
cold sores	lasúlceras de la boca
constipation	el estreñimiento
convulsion	la convulsión
cough	la tos
cramps	los calambres
deafness	la sordera
diabetes	la diabetes
diarrhea	la diarrea
discharge	el flujo
dizziness	el vértigo, el mareo
eczema	el eccema
emphysema	el enfisema
epilepsy	la epilepsia
fainting spell	el desmayo
fatigue	la fatiga
fever	la fiebre
flu	la influenza, la gripe
food poisoning	el envenenamiento por comestibles
fracture	la fractura
gallbladder attack	el ataque de la vesícula biliar

English-Spanish quick reference guide
(continued)

gallstone	el cálculo biliar
gastric ulcer	la úlcera gástrica
glaucoma	el glaucoma
gonorrhea	la gonorrea
headache	el dolor de cabeza
heart attack	el ataque al corazón
heartbeat	el latido
– irregular	irregular
– rhythmical	– rítmico
– slow	– lento
– fast (tachycardia)	– taquicardia
heartburn	las agruras (el ardor), acedía
heart disease	la enfermedad del corazón
heart failure	el fallo cardíaco
heart murmur	el soplo del corazón
hemorrhage	la hemorragia
hemorrhoids	las almorranas, las hemorroides
hepatitis	la hepatitis
hernia	la hernia
herpes	el herpes
high blood pressure	la presión alta
hives	la urticaria
hoarseness	la ronquera
ill	enfermo(a)
illness	la enfermedad
immunization	la inmunización
infarct	el infarto
infection	la infección
inflammation	la inflamación
injury	el daño la lastimadura, la herida
itch	la picazón, la comezón
jaundice	la piel amarilla, la ictericia
kidney stone	el cálculo en el riñón, la piedra en el riñón
laryngitis	la laringitis
lesion	la lesión, el daño
leukemia	la leucemia

(continued)

English-Spanish quick reference guide
(continued)

lice	los piojos
lump	el bulto
malignancy	el tumor, la malignidad
malignant	maligno(a)
measles	el sarampión
meningitis	la meningitis
menopause	la menopausia
metastasis	la metástasis
migraine	la migraña, la jaqueca
multiple sclerosis	la esclerosis múltiple
mumps	las paperas
muscular dystrophy	la distrofia muscular
mute	mudo(a)
obese	obeso(a)
overdose	la sobredosis
overweight	el sobrepeso
pain	el dolor
– growing pain	– el dolor de crecimiento
– labor pain	– el dolor de parto
– phantom limb pain	– el dolor de miembro fantasma
– referred pain	– el dolor referido
– sharp pain	– el dolor agudo
– shooting pain	– el dolor punzante
– burning pain	– el dolor que arde
– intense pain	– el dolor intenso
– severe pain	– el dolor severo
– intermittent pain	– el dolor intermitente
– throbbing pain	– el dolor palpitante
palpitation	la palpitación
paralysis	la parálisis
Parkinson's disease	la enfermedad de Parkinson
pneumonia	la pulmonía
psoriasis	la psoriasis
pus	el pus
rash	la roncha, el salpullido, la erupción
relapse	la recaída
renal	renal

English-Spanish quick reference guide

(continued)

rheumatic fever	la fiebre reumitáca
roseola	la roséola
rubella	la rubéola
rupture	la ruptura
scab	la costra
scar	la cicatriz
scratch	el rasguño
senile	senil
shock	el choque
sore	la llaga
spasm	el espasmo
sprain	la torcedura
stomachache	el dolor del estómago
stomach ulcer	la úlcera del estómago
suicide	el suicidio
swelling	la hinchazón
syphilis	la sífilis
tachycardia	la taquicardia
toothache	el dolor de muela
toxemia	la toxemia
trauma	el trauma
tuberculosis	la tuberculosis
tumor	el tumor
ulcer	la úlcera
unconsciousness	la pérdida del conocimiento
virus	el virus
vomit	el vómito, los vómitos
wart	la verruga
weakness	la debilidad
wheeze	el jadeo, la silba
wound	la herida
yellow fever	la fiebre amarilla

English-Spanish medication administration

I would like to give you:	Quisiera darle a Ud. un(a):
• an injection.	• inyección.
• an I.V. medication.	• medicamento por vía intravenosa.
• a liquid medication.	• medicamento en forma líquida.
• a medicated cream or powder.	• medicamento en pomada o polvo.
• a medication through your epidural catheter.	• medicamento por el catéter epidural.
• a medication through your rectum.	• medicamento por el recto.
• a medication through your _____ tube.	• medicamento por su _____ tubo.
• a medication under your tongue.	• medicamento debajo de la lengua.
• some pill(s).	• píldoras.
• a suppository.	• supositorio.

This is how you take this medication.	Así se toma este medicamento.

If you can't swallow this pill, I can crush it and mix it in some food or liquid such as:	Si Ud. no se puede tragar esta píldora, puedo aplastarla y mezclarla en un alimento/líquido, tal como:
• applesauce.	• puré de manzana.
• pudding.	• pudín.
• yogurt.	• yogur.

If you can't swallow this pill, I can get it in another form.	Si Ud. no puede tragarse esta píldora, puede obtenerla en otra forma.

If you can't swallow a pill, you can crush it and mix it in soft food.	Si Ud. no se puede tragar la píldora, la puede moler y mezclarla en un alimento blando.

I need to mix this medication in juice or water.	Tengo que mezclar este medicamento en jugo (zumo) o agua.

English-Spanish medication administration
(continued)

I need to give you this injection in your:	Tengo que ponerle esta inyección:
• abdomen.	• en el abdomen.
• buttocks.	• en las nalgas.
• hip.	• en la cadera.
• outer arm.	• en el brazo
• thigh.	• en el muslo.

I need to give you this medication I.V.	Tengo que darle este medicamento por vía intravenosa (I.V.).

Place it under your tongue.	Póngaselo debajo de la lengua.

You should feel some burning when it is under your tongue.	Ud. debiera sentir un ardor cuando se lo pone debajo de la lengua.

This indicates that it is working.	Esto indica que está tomando efecto.

Some medications are coated with a special substance to protect your stomach from getting upset.	Algunos medicamentos están cubiertos con una sustancia especial para protegerle contra un trastorno estomacal.

Do not chew:	No masque Ud.:
• enteric-coated pills.	• píldoras con recubrimientoentérico.
• long-acting pills.	• píldoras de efecto prolongado.
• capsules.	• cápsulas.
• sublingual medication.	• medicamentos sublinguales.

English-Spanish medication history

Do you take any medications?	**¿Toma Ud. medicamentos?**
Prescription?	¿De receta?
Over-the-counter?	¿Sin necesidad de receta?
Other?	¿Otro?
Which prescription medications do you take routinely?	**¿Qué medicamentos de receta toma Ud. por rutina?**
How often do you take them?	¿Con qué frecuencia los toma?
Once daily?	¿Una vez al día?
Twice daily?	¿Dos veces al día?
Three times daily?	¿Tres veces al día?
Four times daily?	¿Cuátro veces al día?
More often?	¿Con más frecuencia?
Which over-the-counter medications do you take routinely?	**¿Qué medicamentos que no necesitan receta toma Ud. por rutina?**
How often do you take them?	¿Con que frecuencia los toma?
Once daily?	¿Una vez al día?
Twice daily?	¿Dos veces al día?
Three times daily?	¿Tres veces al día?
Four times daily?	¿Cuatro veces al día?
More often?	¿Con más frecuencia?
Which medications do you take periodically?	**¿Qué medicamentos toma Ud. periódicamente?**
Why do you take these medications?	¿Por qué toma Ud. estos medicamentos?
What is the dosage for each medication?	¿Cuál es la dosis para cada uno de los medicamentos?
How does each medication make you feel?	¿Cómo le hace sentirse cada medicamento?
Are you allergic to any medications?	**¿Está Ud. alérgico(a) a algúnos medicamentos?**
Which medications?	¿A qué medicamentos?
What happens when you have an allergic reaction?	¿Qué pasa cuando Ud. tiene una reacción alérgica?

Dangerous abbreviations

The Joint Commission on the Accreditation of Healthcare Organizations has approved the following "minimum list" of dangerous abbreviations, acronyms, and symbols. Using this list should help protect patients from the effects of miscommunication in clinical documentation.

Abbreviation	Potential problem	Preferred term
U (for unit)	Mistaken as zero, four, or cc	Write "unit"
IU (for international unit)	Mistaken as IV (intravenous) or 10 (ten)	Write "international unit"
Q.D., QD, q.d., qd (daily) Q.O.D., QOD, q.o.d., qod (every other day)	Mistaken for each other; the period after the Q can be mistaken for an "I"; the "O" can also be mistaken for an "I"	Write "daily" or "every other day"
Trailing zero (X.0 mg) (*Note:* Prohibited only for medication-related notations), lack of leading zero (.X mg)	Decimal point is missed	Never write a zero by itself after a decimal point (X mg), and always use a zero before a decimal point (0.X mg)
MS, MSO$_4$, MgSO$_4$	Confused for one another; can mean morphine sulfate or magnesium sulfate	Write "morphine sulfate" or "magnesium sulfate"

Treatment for biological weapons exposure

Listed below are potentially threatening biological (bacterial and viral) agents as well as treatments and vaccines currently available.

Implement standard precautions for all cases of suspected exposure. For smallpox, institute airborne precautions for the duration of the illness and until all scabs fall off. For pneumonic plague cases, institute droplet precautions for 72 hours after initiation of effective therapy.

Biological agent (condition)	Treatment
Bacillus anthracis (anthrax)	• Ciprofloxacin, doxycycline, penicillin • Vaccine: Limited supply available; not recommended in absence of exposure to anthrax
Clostridium botulinum (botulism)	• Supportive; endotracheal intubation and mechanical ventilation • Passive immunization with equine antitoxin to lessen nerve damage • Vaccine: Postexposure prophylaxis with equine botulinum antitoxin; botulinum toxoid available from Centers for Disease Control and Prevention; recombinant vaccine under development
Francisella tularensis (tularemia)	• Gentamicin or streptomycin; alternatively, doxycycline, chloramphenicol, and ciprofloxacin • Vaccine: Live, attenuated vaccine currently under investigation and review by the Food and Drug Administration (FDA)
Variola major (smallpox)	• No FDA-approved antiviral available; cidofovir may be therapeutic if administered 1 to 2 days after exposure • Vaccine: Prophylaxis within 3 to 4 days of exposure
Yersinia pestis (pneumonic plague)	• Streptomycin or gentamicin; alternatively, doxycycline, ciprofloxacin, or chloramphenicol • Vaccine: No longer available

Notes

Notes

Notes

Selected references

American Heart Association. *Handbook of Emergency Cardiovascular Care for Healthcare Providers, 2004 Update.* Dallas: American Heart Association, 2004.

Assessment Made Incredibly Easy, 3rd edition. Philadelphia: Lippincott Williams & Wilkins, 2005.

Braunwald, E., et al. *Harrison's Principles of Internal Medicine,* 16th edition. New York: McGraw Hill, 2005.

ECG Interpretation: An Incredibly Easy Pocket Guide. Philadelphia: Lippincott Williams & Wilkins, 2006.

Fast Facts for Nurses. Philadelphia: Lippincott Williams & Wilkins, 2004.

Fischbach, F.T. *A Manual of Laboratory and Diagnostic Tests,* 7th ed. Philadelphia: Lippincott Williams & Wilkins, 2004.

Handbook of Geriatric Nursing Care. Philadelphia: Lippincott Williams & Wilkins, 2003.

Infusion Nurses Society, Inc. "Infusion Nursing Standards of Practice," *Journal of Intravenous Nursing* (Supplement) 23(6S):S1-S85, November/December 2000.

Masoorli, S., and Angeles, T. "Getting a Line on Central Venous Access Devices," *Nursing2002* 32(4):36-47, April 2002.

NANDA Nursing Diagnoses: 2005-2006: Definitions and Classification. Philadelphia: North American Nursing Diagnosis Association, 2005.

Nursing Procedures, 4th ed. Philadelphia: Lippincott Williams & Wilkins, 2004.

Strickland, O. "Cultural Considerations and Issues in Measurement," *Journal of Nursing Measurement* 11(1)3-4, Spring-Summer 2003.

Wong, D., et al. *Maternal Child Nursing Care,* 3rd edition. Philadelphia: Mosby, 2006.

Index

Resource